For you,
your family,
your dear friends,
your students.

„People really like this book – it works well for people who have never heard of Feldenkrais, because the explanations focus on the important aspects that people need to know. The book really helps people grasp how and why the FM is different from other modalities, how intelligent, effective and unique it is. And the book works equally well for people who know and have experienced the Feldenkrais Method before.

Everyone tells me that they find the book fun, interesting and easy to read and use. They love the pictures and the dialog bubbles. And the book makes it so easy for people to show to their friends and relatives, to explain what it is that they are doing, rather than having to describe, explain or illustrate what the Feldenkrais Method is. They can just hand them the book and say 'Here. This is what I am doing!'

The book is contemporary, user-friendly, has a high quality feel and look; and although it is small, it is packed with info. This book has made a huge difference in my ability to promote and support Feldenkrais in my trade area (or anywhere for that matter), and I am so really glad to have found it as a resource. I hope it will not go out of print!"
– Carole Bucher, GCFP

„Excellent book on the Feldenkrais method, which gives students a very creative perspective."
– Gail T.

„Alfons has created many educational pathways to understanding the Feldenkrais Method of Somatic Education, through his book, his communication skills and opening a very accessible and successful practice. Although I have never experienced his hands, I look forward to someday; and would not hesitate to refer anyone to him for his expertise and knowledge in educating the whole person, and finding a pathway out of pain and towards a satisfying life."
– Deborah Elizabeth Lotus, GCFP

„Easy and immediate"
– Shira S.

„Novel pictorial approach and cool design. Complex information is presented in a clear, simple format that is enjoyable to read. It is aimed at people who are new to the Feldenkrais Method, but I think its refreshing simplicity and clarity also make it a valuable tool for those experienced in the Method. The first part of the book explores some of the concepts underpinning the Feldenkrais Method, and the second part contains several photo stories – presented in a cartoon style, which illustrate some movement explorations. These photo stories are probably the highlight of the book, and I've noticed that when I've shown people the book, it's this section which they are drawn to and become absorbed in."
– Karol

„It's one of the best things I've seen in ages. For everyone who has ever said to me: When my friends ask me what we do in class, and I just can't describe it, this book says it all, plus gives you lessons to play with at home. And I love the Kindle edition which let's you zoom in on the pics!"
– Lavinia Plonka, GCFP

„This is a book to read, study, and go back to again and again. Hope he writes more!"
– Marcia H. Schoppik, GCFP

„This is a very readable guide to the Feldenkrais Method, with clear explanations, directions, and movement exploration sequences. It answers many questions that people have about what to expect in a Feldenkrais class and provides opportunities to experience the benefits of the work in the privacy of their homes if they're not yet able to locate a class near them and to re-enforce the learning from their group lessons if they are Feldenkrais students taking public classes. Plus, the photo sequences are a big help in clarifying the instructions for movement explorations for those whose primary learning modality isn't the written word."
– Sanfeld

„Very clear, concrete, useful manual. Should be put out as a little red book – except about the freedoms the Feldenkrais Method gives us."
– Renée Dunham, GCFP

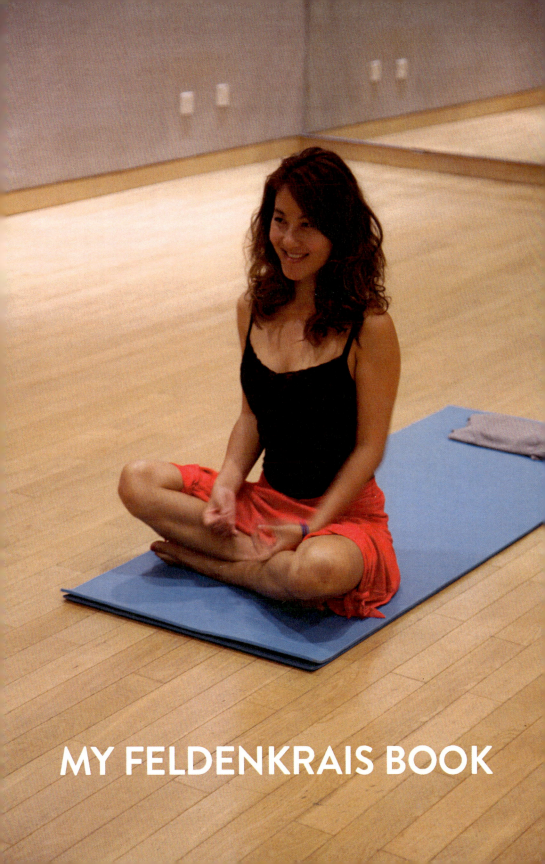

MY FELDENKRAIS BOOK

"My Feldenkrais Book" written by Alfons Grabher
Copyright © Alfons Grabher, All rights reserved.
www.myfeldenkraisbook.com
alfonsgrabher@hotmail.com
6900 Bregenz, Austria, Europe

Please contact me for bulk ordering options.

1st edition November 2010
Edited by Heidi Woehrle
Photo stories photography © Maverick Stoklosa
Type set and print ready by Zeughaus
www.zeughaus.com

2nd edition December 2015 (Version 1, December 2015)
Book design and layout by Alfons Grabher

Feldenkrais Method® is the registered trademark in the U.K. of the Feldenkrais Guild UK Ltd., Reg No. 1563759. Feldenkrais®, Feldenkrais Method®, Functional Integration®, Awareness Through Movement®, and Guild Certified Feldenkrais Practitioner[cm] are service marks in the United States of the FELDENKRAIS GUILD® of North America.

Legal Disclaimer: The information in this book is given in good faith and strictly for reference only and is neither intended to diagnose any physical or mental condition nor to serve as a substitute for medical advice or professional health care. Please remember that no practice can be adequately learned from written descriptions. All Feldenkrais® lessons in this book are designed to complement instruction by a Guild Certified Feldenkrais Practitioner[cm]. Talk to your doctor before starting any new exercise regime.

Printed by Createspace, an Amazon.com company
ISBN-13: 978-1519469199
ISBN-10: 1519469195

TABLE OF CONTENTS

Do I think the Feldenkrais Method is important?	9
A little something about the Feldenkrais Method	13
No workout, no cardio	19
No stretching	19
No drills	20
Respecting individuality	22
To correct is incorrect	23
12 people, 12 different ways	26
Following legs and a twist	29
Establishing, maintaining, and dropping connections – within yourself	34
Learning to let go, literally	34
Feeling differences	35
Elongating arm for back, neck, and shoulders	36
Play with movement initiation	46
Rolling the head	48
Knowledge and knowing	50
The journey is the reward	52
Employ your muscles to their best purpose	53
Trust in self-organization	54
Look beyond habits	55
Resolving the red light reflex	56
Resolving the green light reflex	64
Find what's interesting	75
Joy through simplicity	75
Explore real movements	76
The flexible spine	78
Learn and explore	86
Less is more, go with easy	87
Use it or lose it	88
Reduce effort, instead of increasing it	89
Spiralling to sit, a classic 4-points lesson	90
Who created this book?	102

PLEASE
LIE DOWN
OR SIT
COMFORTABLY

Do I think the Feldenkrais Method is important?

When I was a youngster of 14 years old, my father brought home one of the first computers available: a VIC 20. Back then nobody really knew what this thing was, what it was used for and why it was supposed to be interesting. I, on the other hand, was super excited: I sensed something big and eagerly started exploring it; I even started writing my own software programs. I exchanged these programs with a friend of mine and we agreed that this was indeed the coolest thing in the world. However, I soon found out that my friend and I were the only people around who thought this was the coolest thing ever. Many of our schoolmates couldn't understand what we are doing; they called us „computer freaks". Why would anyone spend their valuable time with an electric typewriter and a blue flickery screen? For them, being „cool" meant drinking beer at the beach and flirting with girls. Nobody had a clue what software was and where it was headed.

All this changed when the first cell phones with tiny screens hit the market. Everybody had to have one. PCs and other computer systems became affordable and began to populate offices and living rooms. People became familiar with „software": it became a key part of daily life.

Nowadays, everyone talks about and relates to software — which programs they like and millions of people buy and download and share software by the dozens each month. People who write iPhone apps or social internet platforms are worshipped like religious leaders. Being a „computer freak" turned into a respectable, well paid profession. Something unknown turned into a popular and indispensable tool that people now can't imagine living without.

I see a similar transformation — from unknown to integral part of society — happening with the Feldenkrais Method. I initially indulged in it because I sensed that there is great value in learning more about oneself. I strongly believe that the principles found in the Feldenkrais Method will be one of society's key drivers following the shift from industrial society to information society. By „learning about oneself" I don't mean just listening to great words of visionaries, best selling writers and motivational gurus (and reflecting on their intriguing thoughts), but actually applying a practical method that gives results. Not just short-lived, subjectively perceived results, but solid, lasting changes for the long-term.

As of now, the Feldenkrais Method appears without a popular face, without celebrity actresses, without singers or gurus promoting it. Without big marketing departments and mind-boggling budgets. Without sexy outfits, healthy drinks, esoteric beats and fancy accessories. Even so, this valuable knowledge has been steadily finding more and more people in the last 50 years. It's spreading because it's profound and it works.

The science behind Feldenkrais lessons is interdisciplinary and closely related to Biology and Human Evolution, Child Development, Cognitive Sciences and Linguistics, Ericksonian Hypnotherapy, Medicine, History and Culture, Neuropsychology, Neuroscience, Psychology, Philosophy, as well as martial arts for self defense.

I'm not sure whether or not the „Feldenkrais Method" will arrive in people's households with this name. The method is remarkably rich, with hundreds of lessons. Maybe it will be served in smaller portions and more easily accessible packages with different names. But it seems obvious that the key concepts will, in one form or another, inevitably arrive in everyone's home.

ABOUT THIS BOOK AND WHY I WROTE IT

Feldenkrais lessons seem to be simple and easy to follow along, but are actually quite rich in content. For me, teaching the Feldenkrais Method is an amazing experience. Seeing people learning about themselves and evolving, taking better care of themselves and becoming younger in appearance is a marvellous view. However, it appears to me that some of my comments during class are lost in time and space. It's also a challenge for some students to discover key concepts in a timely manner. Therefore I wanted to give my students something solid, something like a book to look up important study points, a companion for group classes.

I want this companion to clarify some key findings; to deepen the students' learning after class. This companion should also explain (a bit at least) why the Feldenkrais Method is a category of its own — for example, how does it differ from other similar-looking modalities (a bunch of people on yoga mats plus a teacher)?

I have the impression that most people come to classes to find relief from pain. But the Feldenkrais Method can be so much more. Therefore, you won't find a concise definition here. Instead, the aim of the book is to give you an impression of what you are dealing with in Feldenkrais classes. And give you some pictures of people doing classic Feldenkrais lessons, which you can show when somebody asks you „what is it people are doing there?". I tried to make this book a pleasant, easy read. It aims to heighten understanding from the students' perspective and focuses on concepts that are directly helpful to improve one's personal practice.

I learned that a book like this could not be done alone: I needed a whole network of people. I want to thank the many people I met through the process of creating this book, people without whom the book would not have been possible:

Maverick Stoklosa for his photography; Stefania, Valeria, Giorgio, Guillaume, Aurora, Sabine and Kenji for being adventurous enough to appear in the photos; huge thanks to Heidi for her editing, greatly helpful comments and positive energy; David @ ufohunter.net for helping me get started with the layout, superhuman huge thanks to Oliver and the team @ zeughaus.com for the final layout editing and making the book print ready — even though they had much pressure from other, much bigger projects they gave me the feeling that this book is their only and most important one; Richard Brown at bodyworksasia.cn for providing a teaching space and many valuable tips; big thanks to Cyril and Nick for providing me with a home during my stays in Hong Kong; the guys from ekohe.com for letting me sit in their office; my previous and current students for everything I learned from them; Big thanks to Michelle for making me come to Taiwan: without the inspiration there I would have never been able to make the photo stories; Bert Hellinger for his permission to use his poem and the version in English he sent me; Elsa, John, Nick, Colin and everyone else for commenting on the book's structure and sentence style.

I hope this book will assist you to understand more about yourself in Feldenkrais classes, and grant you deeper access to the marvellous, rejuvenating physical, emotional, and mental benefits that you are thus able to experience. Enjoy.

NOTES ON THE 2ND EDITION

To write a book is one thing. To show it to people and sell it, another. I would like to thank everyone who helped with the second, much more daunting task. It's much easier for students to find good reads when they get recommendations from their teachers. In this sense a big „Thank you" to Carole Bucher, Jenni Evans, and Suellen Bartel, my biggest supporters I know of – sharing is caring. If you like this book, please help telling others about it (and also tell me, I love to hear good feedback).

It's been five years, and almost all copies of the 1st edition have been sold. I was asked to not have it go out of print. Therefore I decided to release a 2nd edition. As you may know, I had the 1st edition printed in China. On one hand printing in China can be cheaper than anywhere else in the world, but it also comes with an up front financial investment, shipping costs, import taxes, storage fees, as well as a long term storage management. Therefore, this time I opted for print on demand with Createspace, an Amazon company. They do a great job with printing and shipping. On the downside printing costs are much higher (more than four times as much), and they require a standard trim-size. Which in turn required a complete rework of the book.

And because I had to move every sentence down to every single letter, every picture, every speech bubble anyway, I decided to update some of the headlines, texts and speech bubbles as well (without diverting from the original ideas). In the time between the 1st and 2nd edition I've been teaching well over 400 group classes, learned a lot, and I just couldn't help to rephrase some of the original writings. It's still the same book, but in a mainstream trim size, completely rearranged layout with just as many pages as absolutely necessary, and extensively updated wording.

A little something about the Feldenkrais Method

Moshé Feldenkrais is the inventor of the Feldenkrais Method. He was born 1904 in the Ukrainian town of Slavuta; deceased in 1984 in Tel Aviv; earned his doctor's degree in Physics at the Sorbonne, Paris; dedicated the entire last third of his life solely to teaching what today is called the Feldenkrais Method. From the plethora of interesting facts in his career, I picked two:

1) In 1933, Moshé Feldenkrais was invited to work in the team of Nobel Prize laureate Frédéric Joliot-Curie at the Curie Institute Sorbonne, Paris. Together they created the first french particle accelerator, a technology needed for atomic energy, medical research and organic chemistry.

2) In 1936, Moshé Feldenkrais became one of the first Europeans to earn a Black Belt in Judo; Judo is a Japanese fighting sport and can be translated as „the gentle way". Still in Paris, Feldenkrais became close friends with Jigaro Kano, the creator of modern Judo. With Kano's support he was a co-founding member of the Jiu Jitsu Club de France, one of the oldest Judo clubs in Europe. It still exists today.

There are two similar patterns in these two seemingly different fields of expertise: small changes in external conditions lead to enormous changes in the will of the actor. Atomic processes start with the collision of tiny particles, and once unleashed lead to chain reaction and the availability of enormous power; in Judo, the players pay close attention to the moves of one another. Small mistakes in balance or stance are amplified and allow for energetic throws to bring down the opponent.

In these methods, small adjustments lead to big change. The same is true for the effects experienced in Feldenkrais lessons. However, these lessons are peaceful and the improvements are for the client's benefit. Many lessons start out with comfortable, easy movements that gradually evolve into movements of greater range and complexity. There are hundreds of lessons that vary from simple to physically demanding. When done attentively, there's no pain or sweat involved. There are two modes of teaching:

a) Individual lessons (officially called „Functional Integration"). Here, lessons are taught one on one. The client lies fully dressed on a table that is somewhat similar to a massage table. Through gentle touch, and careful push and pull, the practitioner communicates with the client in a non-verbal fashion. While the practitioner is doing most of the work, the client's job is to follow the moves attentively.

b) Group classes (officially called „Awareness Through Movement" or in short, „ATM"). Here, several people come together for a class. These classes may be structured quite similar to individual lessons, but have hardly any hands-on guidance. Students are guided verbally through movement sequences. In this way, everyone is encouraged to move independently.

Even though Moshé Feldenkrais, the inventor of the Feldenkrais Method, doesn't live any longer, his teachings are as actual and unmatched in genius as thirty years ago.

However, many Feldenkrais Practitioners do not stick strictly to the Feldenkrais trademark and Moshe Feldenkrais's lectures, notes, and transcripts: they teach and market their own brands. Just for example: Bones for Life™, a program for building bone tissue via natural movement. Hanna Somatic Education® a system of neuromuscular education (mind-body training) which helps to enjoy freedom from pain and more comfortable movement. Cure TMJ, simple Feldenkrais self-care practices for easing TMJ symptoms. The Dynamic Musician Series, lessons intended to improve sound quality and musical performance. The Effortless Swing, lessons designed to bring every golfer back to natural, easy movements, and many more. As unique as these programs are, they all rely on the very principles taught in Feldenkrais classes.

WHY DO PEOPLE COME TO CLASSES?

The Feldenkrais Method has a large variety of lessons. Newcomers to the Feldenkrais Method mostly search for a way to resolve conditions related to musculoskeletal pain (e.g. knee problems, lower back pain, neck tension, disc herniation). However, these applications are just the beginning. Removing pain and recovering function, as profound as these may appear, only set the basic conditions for continuous improvement. Consequently, lessons will also improve a person's general movement quality, ability to feel, sense, as well as perceive oneself and others.

Apart from the quantifiable benefits, Feldenkrais classes make students feel comfortable, at ease, peaceful. The movement sequences themselves keep surprising and inspiring students with their finesse and ingenuity. Here's a selection of things students say about Feldenkrais classes:

Carriage of the head (where 4 out of 5 senses are located) improves; shorter time needed to fall asleep; better coordination in rock climbing; Strength of grip increases; Appearance of being younger, better skin tonus; fewer concerns about „small" things; Less distress about disturbances; reduction of work related stress; reduction of neck tension; relief from lower back pain; Learning efficiency improves; Ability to concentrate improves; Ability to enjoy movement and life as a whole increases; Find harmony and healing; More flexibility for mind and body; improved balance and motor skills; fluidity and ease of movement; Improvement of motor control and refined movement; Increased flexibility of spine; More energy, less fatigue; Gastrointestinal function normalizes; Having more options in life; Fewer headaches; Ability to relax improves; Better sleep; Eye-hand coordination improves; More positive feelings about self; Improvement in overall health, general well-being and experience of quality of life; Attention improves; fewer angry outbursts; become more aware of your body's posture, alignment and patterns of movement; Well-being increases; less depression and more interest in life; Range of motion increase; decreased moodiness; Mood improves and subjective well-being increases; Habitual tension decreases; Pain decreases; Depth perception improves; Spatial awareness increases; Kinesthetic sense improves; Balance improves; Anxiety and Depression decrease; Self-acceptance and self-actualization increase; awareness of personal life improves; Ability to adapt to change improves; Decreased hostility; Tolerance of dysfunctional relationships decreases; physical appearance and radiance improves; feel fitter, be more energetic, happier and peaceful; Mood improves; Concentration improves; Improves posture, flexibility, function, and coordination; Reduces stress and increases self-confidence; Eases chronic pain and movement restrictions; Helps overcome and avoid injuries; refined skills for athletes, musicians and dancers; Softer, more healthy looking skin; Improved posture in sitting, standing and walking; Relief of pain and ability recover from and prevent injury; Increased capacity to benefit from other alternative therapies; Increased strength, endurance, and energy; Improved flexibility, balance and coordination; Greater self-awareness and self-satisfaction; Reduce anxiety and stress; Achieve restful sleep; Reverse pains and limitations of the aging process; Enhanced performance in music, dance, theatre, and athletics; Access to creative thinking and problem solving; Ability to change habits in many areas of life; Improved relationship with yourself and others; more healthy, powerful, easy and pleasurable exertion; reduction of tension; more efficient, effortless movement; greater awareness of inefficiency and effort; gradual reduction of useless effort; Increased kinesthetic sensitivity, better self regulation; more self-knowledge and awareness of own doings; early return to sport; improved quality of life... and much more.

SPREAD

In 1954, Dr. Moshé Feldenkrais started teaching his method full-time in Tel Aviv/Israel. Later he was invited to lecture and teach in many renowned institutions all over the world, including France, England, Germany, USA, Switzerland, even in Japan. Nowadays, Feldenkrais classes thought by certified Feldenkrais teachers (aka „Feldenkrais Practitioners") are available just about everywhere. Regular classes are held in more than 30 countries and 10 languages. Class sizes range from as small as 1 person to well over 200 people.

There is quite a large number of resources available on the Feldenkrais Method. Moshé Feldenkrais himself has written seven books on the method, as well as a whole range of articles. Currently, over 100 books about the Feldenkrais Method are available.

Many of the written publications contain lesson instructions. But there are also books with case studies and theoretical reflections. And now there's also two long awaited biographies on Moshé Feldenkrais available: „A Life in Movement – The Biography of Moshé Feldenkrais" by Mark Reese, and on a separate account, the biography in German language „Moshé Feldenkrais – Der Mensch hinter der Methode" by Christian Buckard.

The Internet, too, has a vast selection of resources available: interviews, articles, blogs, podcasts, home study products and free audio lessons. On PubMed (U.S. National Library of Medicine) 30+ scientific studies about various aspects of the Feldenkrais Method can be found. There's also plenty of lessons available from a wide variety of Feldenkrais teachers via youtube, in MP3 format, on CD and DVD.

However, the most practical and efficient way to study the Feldenkrais Method is directly from a Guild certified Feldenkrais Practitioner. Depending on individual needs, one can choose between group classes and private lessons. Lessons are usually taught in rented community space, dedicated Feldenkrais venues, private homes, hospitals, Yoga studios, Pilates studios, Gyms, or Universities (e. g. London Metropolitan University, University of Utah, Music Conservatory of Bern, University of Art/Buenos Aires).

DIFFERENCES TO OTHER METHODS

No workout, no cardio

There are no static workout routines, fixed reps sets, or cardio exercises in Feldenkrais lessons. Moreover, there is no focus on improving VO_2 max scores („VO_2 max" is the maximum rate of oxygen consumption as measured during incremental exercise, most typically on a motorized treadmill). In this way, the Feldenkrais Method is not in the same category with cardio workout, modern postural Yoga, Pilates, Crossfit or similar sports focusing on aesthetics, strength and cardio fitness.

We are made from flesh and blood, and therefore many of us love a good workout. But each one of us also has the most complex, most mysterious and most plastic organ ever found on this planet built in: the human central nervous system.

The benefits experienced with Feldenkrais lessons are achieved through learning more about oneself, making good use of one's cognitive capabilities and working the plasticity of the central nervous system – as opposed to merely strengthening muscles and building up red blood cell count. The Feldenkrais Method is an educational system. There's a strong emphasis on creating a learning environment: a certain atmosphere that promotes exploration and creativity during classes.

No stretching

There are no stretching exercises in Feldenkrais classes, in the sense that muscles are pulled against resistance. In this regard there is no warm-up stretching, no cool-down stretching, no hold-the-posture stretching; no static, dynamic, nonballistic, AIS, not even PNF stretching. Such stretching methods are not part of the Feldenkrais Method.

However, after Feldenkrais lessons most students experience an increased range of motion, ease of movement, and suppleness; all without any muscle soreness our fatigue. How is that possible?

Every lesson, besides having a wide range of benefits, leads the student towards gaining enough range of motion to be able to perform daily activities without restraint. The less physical and mental force is applied, the greater the results. The increased range of motion (without stretching) could come as a result of various improvements: better internal body organization („better organization" is a Feldenkrais concept), a lower muscle resting tonus, yet at the same time being more ready for movement, a more harmonious timing of the opening and closing of various joints, various synergy effects (e. g. relaxing the neck muscles will also relax the hamstring muscles), or maybe other causes altogether? Feldenkrais very obviously works, but there's still a lot of research that needs to be done to be able to understand *how* it works.

On that note: James Stephens did a study on hamstring lengthening, called „Lengthening the Hamstring Muscles Without Stretching Using Awareness Through Movement", published in Physical Therapy, Journal of the American Physical Therapy Association (PHYS THER. 2006; 86:1641-1650). The study comes to following conclusion: „We have shown that hamstring muscles can be lengthened by a method (The Feldenkrais Method) that does not involve stretching."

No drills

In Feldenkrais classes students repeat movements several times. Usually somewhere between 5, 10 or even up to 25 times, depending on how long students can focus (or find something interesting). Rather than mechanically executing a movement exactly the same way over and over again according to a predefined number of reps each, it's left to the student and to every moment when to continue and when to stop.

Moreover, an important focus is to learn more about the movement at hand with each repetition. This might still be uncommon in many fitness exercises for the hobbyist, but not so for the elite sportsman. For example, George Liset, a coach for men's and women's throwing events at the University of New Hampshire, writes on his blog: „The 2004 Olympic gold medalist in the hammer throw Koji Murofushi (JPN), who is at 1.87 m and 90 kg, is one of the lightest and slimmest world-class performers in the event. However, Murofushi's technique makes up for his relative lack of physical presence and with this he has achieved a personal best of 84.86 m, making him the 5th ranked thrower of all time.

Some say Murofushi's technique was inherited from his father Shigenobu, who was a five time Asian Games champion and held the Japanese national record in the event until his son captured it in 1998. The younger Murofushi's ability to control movement has been developed through many years of training and a countless number of throws. Commenting on his technique and his ability to chase the perfect throw, he has said: 'You have to adjust yourself for every attempt taking consideration of many factors in the field. Not a single throw should be the same as any other one.'

What are some of the factors and considerations that go into developing a kinesthetic sense so refined as to be able to throw at an elite level?"

As George Liset's example shows, there is a distinct approach to master certain techniques in sports. While the hobbyist tries to figure out an ultimate one-for-all technique and tries to get closer towards this one goal with mere force and repetition, the elite sportsman goes for variations. This key point is revealed in the statement, „Not a single throw should be the same as any other one." However, variations must be minimal, and one's motor skills must be well enough developed to distinguish among such minimal differences. It's a circle reference: on one end it's the kinesthetic sense that must be able to sense the minimal differences produced by the very same human being on the other end. Playing with his increasingly refined abilities, the elite sportsman gains far more knowledge and experience than the hobbyist. Thus, he is able to instantly react and adjust his technique to the constant variation of given factors in the field. These factors mustn't necessarily be internal, but can also include weather conditions, equipment, or peer pressure.

In Feldenkrais classes it is recommended to take a short break in between each move and then start afresh. Students try to maintain awareness of their movements. Once the awareness is lost, learning no longer takes place. When this stage is reached, a new movement is introduced and a new set of „repetitions" begins. In this way, movements are kept fresh and interesting – as if doing them for the first time. In Feldenkrais lessons repetitions are not like the repetitions in fitness exercises, but are explorations and variations of movement.

Respecting individuality

We identify our loved ones, friends, people we like or have frequent contact with not only by their face, voice, or smell, but also by the way they walk and move. We can spot such a person from a distance.

Technically, this is due to differences in the back, the hips, the knees, the ankles; how people hold their neck, how they move their shoulders and hips, variety in gait, etc. However the world is not that technical.

The way a person moves is just about who they are. As Feldenkrais Method practitioners we look at the whole person, and we don't try to strip off individuality. We don't try to change a person into this or that. There's no dress code and no enforced ideal of looks or posture or how to sit or stand or hold one's head.

There is no competition in how deep one can go into a posture or movement, or how benevolent or „good" someone behaves or is considered by others. There's no intent of preventing a person from engaging to „not-so-aesthetic" looking moves or to repress feelings or thoughts. Nor is there encouragement for these things.

In Feldenkrais classes we approve of a person as who this person is, and we try to show variations and choices. We don't blame someone for what others would perceive as not good or wrong (e. g. if one shoulder appears to be higher than the other, if someone holds his/her head in a pecking position, if some muscles are too weak, if someone slouches while sitting, if a posture is not in alignment with a school or technique, or if someone's breathing appears to be too deep or too shallow or in the wrong places, etc). Instead we enable a person to notice what is possible for her/himself and acknowledge that a person is always trying to move to the best of her/his ability. It's called „The Feldenkrais Method of Somatic Education", we attend to learn and play, explore and discover, evolve and elaborate, instead of being molded, disciplined and adjusted.

To correct is incorrect

Students trying to copy a teacher and a teacher trying to correct students is common almost everywhere; even in activities that call for awareness like Yoga, Tai Chi, dance or music. In many cases, the master is external and absolute; the students then try to follow and copy the external source as accurately as possible.

In Feldenkrais classes, however, there is hardly any correcting. Nor are there lengthy demonstrations.

Corrections (if any) happen mostly in beginner classes to comfort students, since many are not yet used to not being corrected. Demos are mainly used for motivational purposes, comfort building, or to give new ideas when students are stuck.

The Feldenkrais practitioner is not an unquestionable authority who will teach the „right" way to move. Instead, his or her job is to help students find the movements — as well as the study points as described later in the book — within themselves and their range of possibilities.

Dr. Moshé Feldenkrais himself spoke extensively about „not correcting" in his method; he exclaimed „our learning is the most important thing we have!" One of his rather prominent pedagogic concepts was to enable students to be able to learn independently from being corrected.

PHOTO STORIES + STUDY POINTS

A question frequently heard by Feldenkrais practitioners is „Can Feldenkrais help me with back pain / knee pain / balance problems / joint stiffness... ?" Part of the answer is „Yes, it can", but there's more to it. Feldenkrais is a method of somatic education and thus has more to offer than „merely" rehabilitation. In fact, it helps the student to become proficient in certain skills, which in turn, will allow him to improve continuously.

Theory is one thing, practice is another. To quote Austrian writer Ernst Ferstl: „The difference between theory and practice is in practice much greater than in theory". There's a difference in just talking about Feldenkrais, and actually attending classes. Feldenkrais classes provide a learning platform; each class is presented in a way that study points can be found and improved continuously. The benefits – freedom from pain, reduced tension, improved motor skills, younger appearance, better sports performance – will emerge as a by-product of learning.

My suggestion is to focus, for a while at least, on the study points mentioned in this chapter, and less on the functions and postures themselves. Of course the movements themselves are highly interesting too. The combinations and variations even more so. Flexion of the torso following an extension, adding a twist and then flexion again... what primal reflexes get triggered? How do postural constraints facilitate movement of otherwise impossible to mobilize joints? How does a change of posture, e. g. from lying supine to lying prone, change the very same movement, e. g. lifting the head? Fascinating biomechanics, pedagogic concepts, neuropsychological connections. However, I want to shift the focus away from such „academic" viewpoints, and more onto quality of movement, or soft skills of movement so to speak, the subtle „study points".

Not all of these study points can be learned at once. Some will be forgotten and found again; some need time to be refined; some are difficult to improve; some build upon others. Most of them get better with practice. „Better" means a deeper understanding, a more profound feel. I list them in no particular order, and intertwined them with the photo stories. Learning situations for specific abilities will emerge in the lessons. A student can either work on a certain study point intentionally, or just wait until improvements come naturally. There are hundreds, maybe well over a thousand distinct lessons in Moshé Feldenkrais's legacy. Let's see how Feldenkrais lessons can look like, for example...

12 people, 12 different ways

Hardly anyone looks like another. The same is true for voice, posture, and even for movement: every person moves as differently compared to everyone else just as they look differently. If you are to ask 12 people to stand their feet (starting from a supine position with legs straight) you will see 12 different ways to do so.

While a paperback book cannot show movement, it can show postures. Even with such a seemingly simple posture as standing the feet while lying supine, we can see differences in people as big as their faces are different.

Which differences can you spot? How close together/far apart are the feet? How far apart is the right/left foot from the pelvis? How much is the right/left foot rotated outwards/inwards? How much is the right/left knee tilted to the outside/inside? Are all toes touching the ground?

When you see this for real, in a Feldenkrais class, you will notice that each person has a different way to guide his feet to standing. Just as everyone has his own, distinctive handwriting. It's very rare to see someone bringing his feet to standing in a completely different way every time they stand their feet, or to see someone having his feet standing in a completely different place every time.

What does this mean? Just like in graphology (the analysis of physical characteristics and patterns of handwriting) we can dare to make assumptions about a person's awareness of himself, habits and tensegrity structure. If the knees are not perfectly poised over the feet, which might just be the case in all 12 examples, then the muscles around the hip joints must be active, tense even. They have to be, because a knee which is not poised over the foot, will undoubtedly fall over to the side. Gravity wants to do its work.

Now it's the Feldenkrais practitioner's task to teach a lesson that is helping students to become aware of unnecessary tension in themselves (be it in their hips, lower backs, their chests and jaws and cheeks and eyes and other areas that might be relevant). To help them find better places to put their feet. To show them alternatives. To help them make better choices and to learn more about themselves.

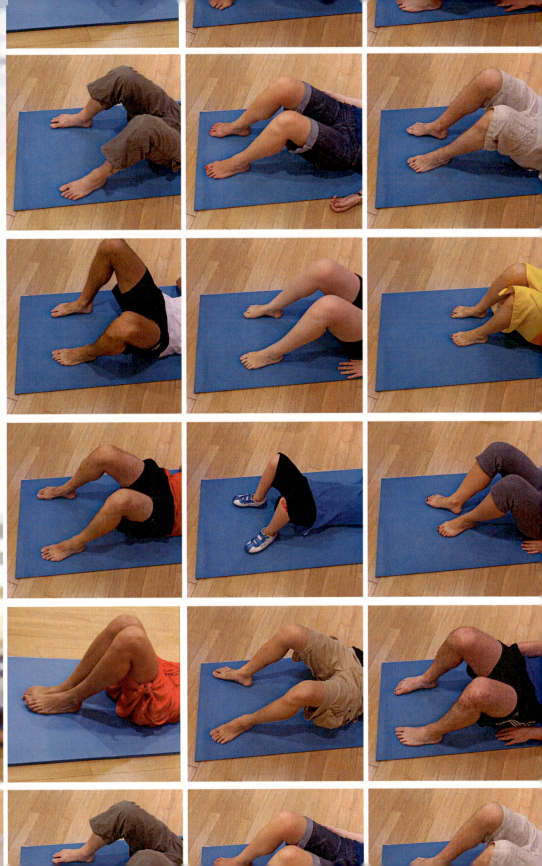

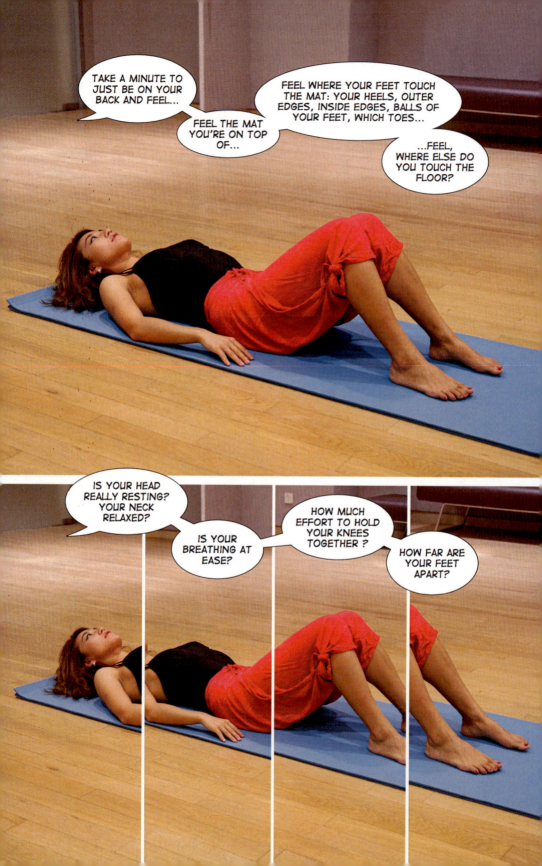

Following legs and a twist

There are hundreds, maybe well over a thousand distinct Feldenkrais lessons. Therefore it's always a bit of a challenge to pick one. In this regard it helps to ask questions like „for what purpose? What do I want to learn?"

With this lesson I want to show how to let go of habitual tension in the hip joints. How to let go, in a literal sense. This will help with having the legs standing with less effort. It will also lead to a very nice feeling around the hip joints, a sort of relaxation and feeling at ease. We will also attempt to transfer this feeling to the chest, neck and shoulders. There's a twist to it: a twist in the torso occurs when the pelvic girdle is rotated in relation to the shoulder girdle (and vice versa). This lesson will enable you to release habitual tension in your chest, and thus be slightly more upright – experiencing a feeling of being taller, more at ease in standing. After such a lesson some women might experience having a bigger „chest", due to a more upright posture.

It is important to go slow in this lesson. Only then you will be able to notice how everything is connected. For the more inflexible students the knee will still be up high when a pull is being felt either on the inside part of the leg, or the other knee. This might be less of a physical constraint, but more of a habitual stress. This lesson is not about stretching, but rather about looking for a feeling of letting go of tension.

Try these movements many times, very slowly. Each time you will find your knee can move a bit further before tension is felt or the other knee lifts. You will feel how your knees are connected.

To prevent the movements from getting boring or inefficient, try pointing your awareness to different spots in your body. For example, just focus on how you roll over the foot, how the weight of your leg shifts from the inside edge of your foot, over the center (also center of heel, and first - second- third - forth - fifth toes, ball of the foot) and the outside edge. Another example would be to just focus on your hip joint. If you can't feel your hip joint, try putting your hand on near your hip joint or upper leg. Just try to sense what's going on inside there. This movement will teach you a lot about your quality of movement in general, as well as how to relax and let go of tension.

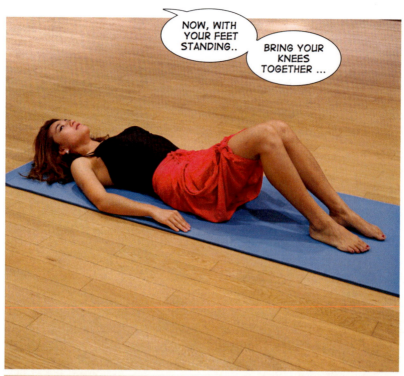

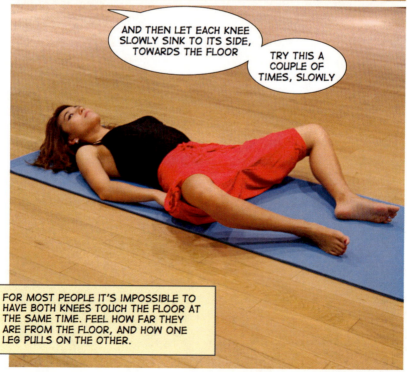

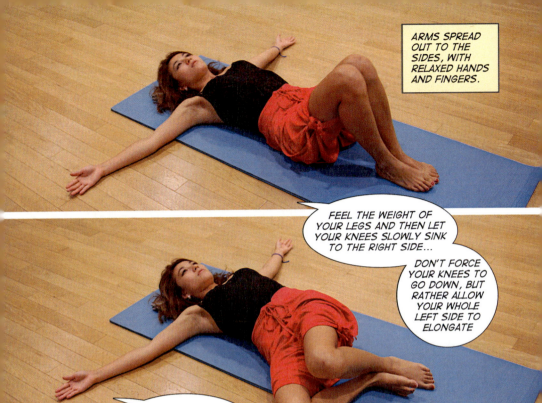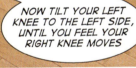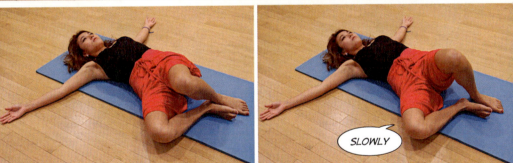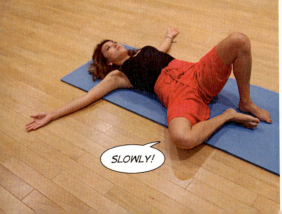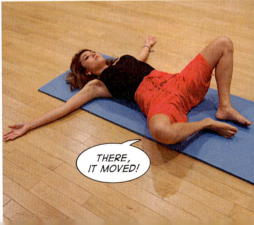

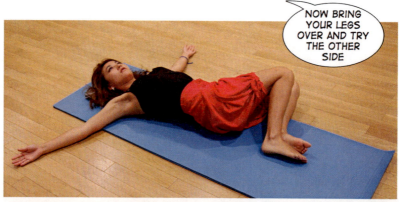
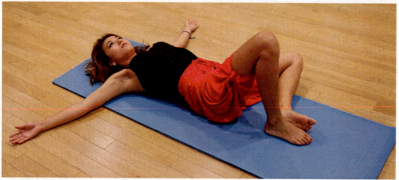
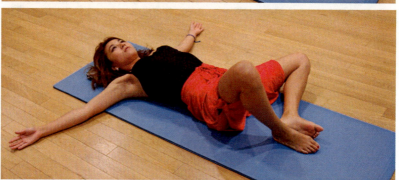
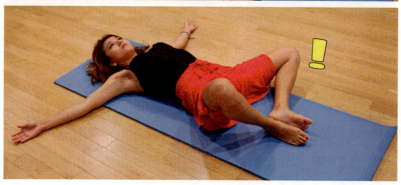

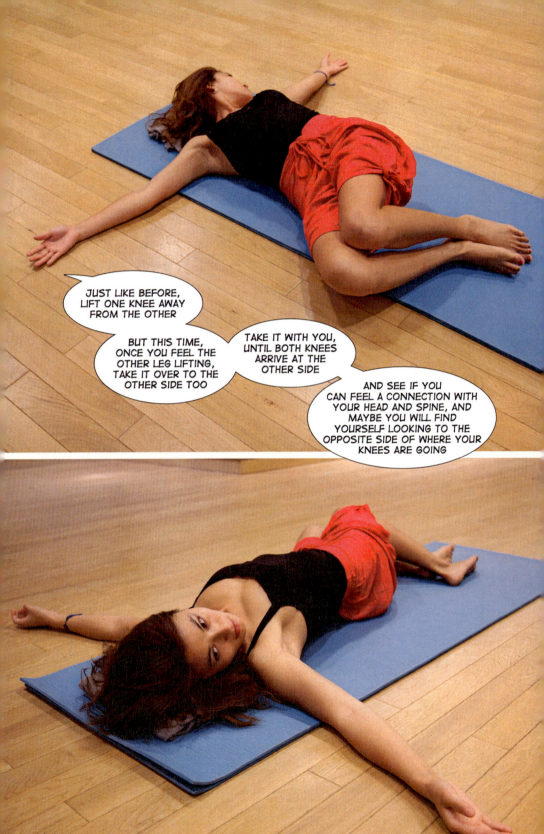

Establishing, maintaining, and dropping connections – within yourself

A human being is made up of parts: hands, arms, shoulders, hips, legs, and so on. All these parts fit together to make up one human being. Even though this is not how a human being is created, this way of thinking has its benefits for finding how the parts are connected.

To give an example: one shoulder can be connected to the other, and lifting one shoulder will affect the other; one leg can be connected to the other leg, and moving one leg will affect the leg on the other side. How this feels and how it actually works is all part of Feldenkrais lessons; here the student has the time and conditions to find and work with these relationships.

Some relationships between body parts seem to be meaningful connections, but on a second look turn out to be arbitrary connections, linked only by habitual patterns in movement, picked up somewhere for some reason — but no longer serve any purpose.

Finding these connections offers a lot of surprises, and sorting out the meaningful from the less supportive ones will provide some of the major benefits that the Feldenkrais Method has to offer. Eventually this will lead to a feeling of being one whole person as opposed to someone assembled from many different parts.

Learning to let go, literally

Everybody knows how to contract muscles. When someone grabs a cup, gets hold of a chair to move it, or pulls on a door — there is contraction. Everybody is familiar with this feeling and can relate to it — using muscle power to contract, flex, extend and twist, to pull or push or squeeze or hold onto something. Less commonly trained, yet equally important, is that muscles can be released. However, this does not refer to the term „extension", performed by extensor-muscles. Just like contraction, releasing and letting go of muscle contractions involves a certain kind of feeling and intention. For many people it seems quite challenging to develop this skill, to find this feeling; and yes, for some it actually takes a while to find it and get better at it.

This seems to be a small thing, but it's a major skill. The ability to let go of tension is essential; for example, letting go of tension in the neck, the jaw, the eyes, the shoulders, in between the ribs of the rib-cage, the hands, the legs, the feet, and so forth. We will find all that in Feldenkrais lessons. Not facilitated by willpower and spoken command, but by clever movement explorations, for example by progressively going into a twist of the entire torso. Feeling, identifying, and differentiating from each other all that can move and twist and turn.

There's entire methods dedicated to just this one thing, on how to let go, how to undo muscle tension; however, here we aren't looking at other methods. It's all neatly built into the Feldenkrais Method. We are exploring what the feeling of letting go feels like, which movements and movement qualities do serve this purpose, and how to let go, literally.

Feeling differences

Even if a movement is repeated several times over, there might still be small differences among repetitions. This is due to our organic nature, due to the fact that we are organic beings — not mechanical robots.

Contrariwise, if a door is opened and closed 500 times, it will (hopefully) open and close in exactly the same way as always. Now consider this movement expoloration: lying on the back, knees extended/legs long, rolling the right leg outwards and inwards. First the toes of the right foot may point towards the ceiling, then to the right side, then towards the ceiling again. Do slow movements, ten times with awareness. Afterwards, the right hip joint will move and feel a tiny bit differently.

Maybe the toes will point to somewhere else than before: more towards the ceiling or more towards the side. Maybe there is a new feeling of relaxation or tension, and it might seem so natural that you think, well, maybe it was already like that. Or perhaps it's not just a little bit easier or lighter; maybe you have the feeling that the right leg seems more „present" than the other. Look for these changes in the photo stories!

However, it's not important what has changed, but the ability to feel that something indeed has changed. That's valuable information for becoming more skillful — at whatever you are seeking improvement.

Elongating arm for back, neck, and shoulders

A Feldenkrais practitioner might argue that every Feldenkrais lesson is equally important, equally well crafted, and provides just as much to learn as any other Feldenkrais lesson. But on a more technical level, lessons differ considerably from each other in terms of structure, content, effect and difficulty.

In this regard, we can almost choose lessons in the same way as a painter chooses a certain brush or colour to achieve a certain effect, or how a doctor chooses a certain medicine to address a certain ailment. This lesson, a twist in side-lying position, elongating and sliding the arm, rolling the head on the floor, would be „prescribed" for any person suffering of a sore neck, restricted range of motion of the head, tension in the shoulders, upper back, or maybe even stiff or sore jaw muscles. There's many more lessons similar to this one, dozens of lessons, no worries... but as a beginning: this is the go to lesson for everything neck pain.

Starting position: on the right side, palms together, elbows straight, hands in front of chest (not in front of nose or belly), shoulders on top of each other (as possible), knees together, ankles together, right angles in hips and knees (as convenient).

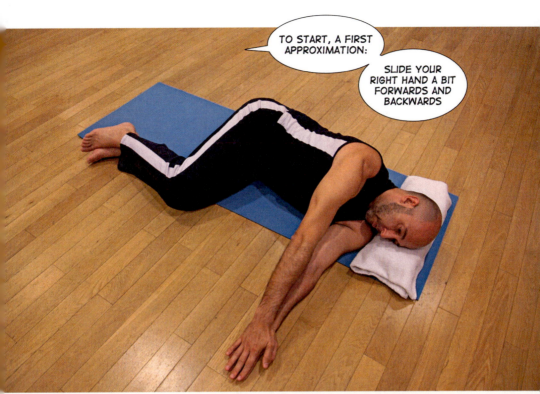
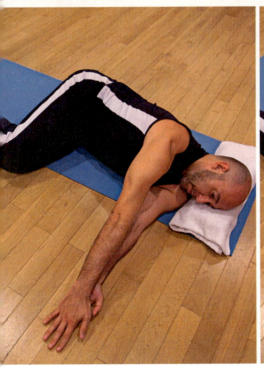
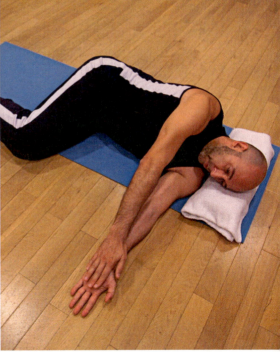

It's not only the shoulder that moves; it's the whole person. The neck, the head, the eyes, the ribs, the belly, the pelvis and knees – each of them moves, and each of them moves in relation to the others. If, as a habit and in daily life, only the shoulder blade moves in isolation (or contrariwise: not at all), then soreness and pain might be the consequence. To get a better sense of what's going on, sometimes it's helpful to have someone else to lend and hand. Or imagine there's another person helping you to discover how all parts can roll, lengthen, participate and support.

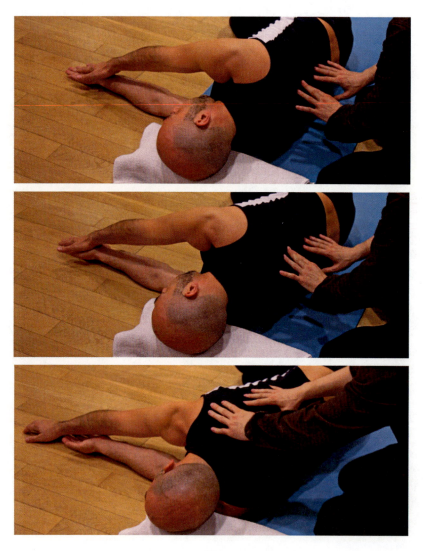

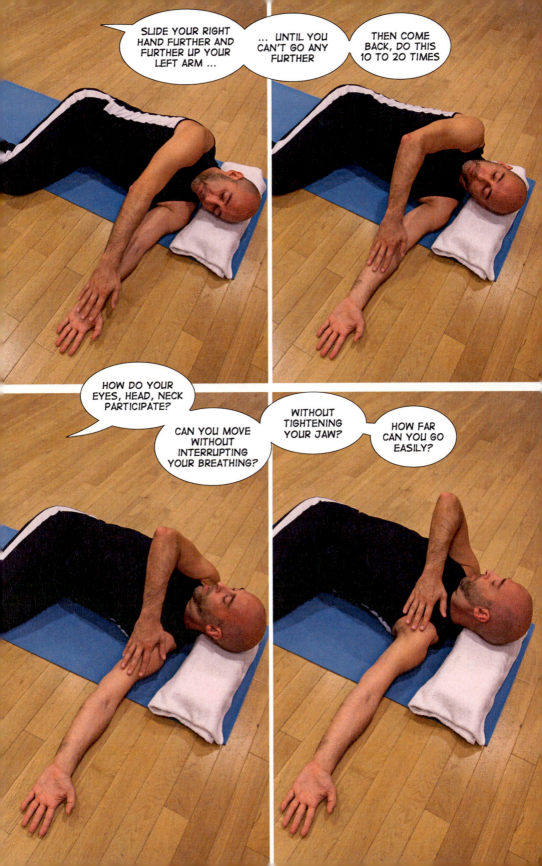

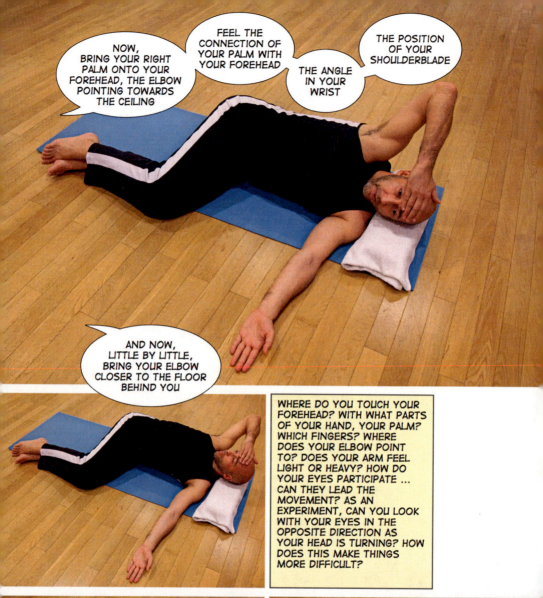
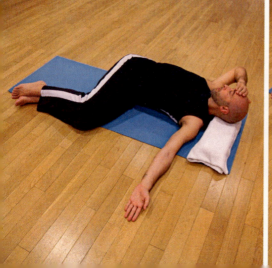
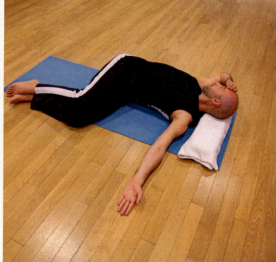

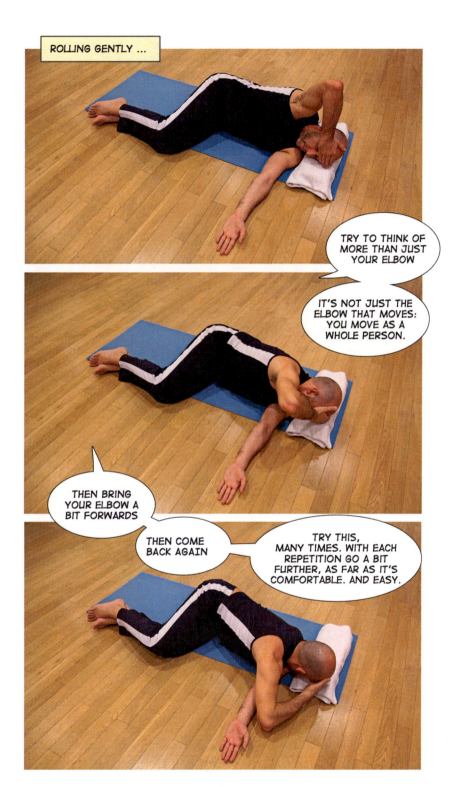

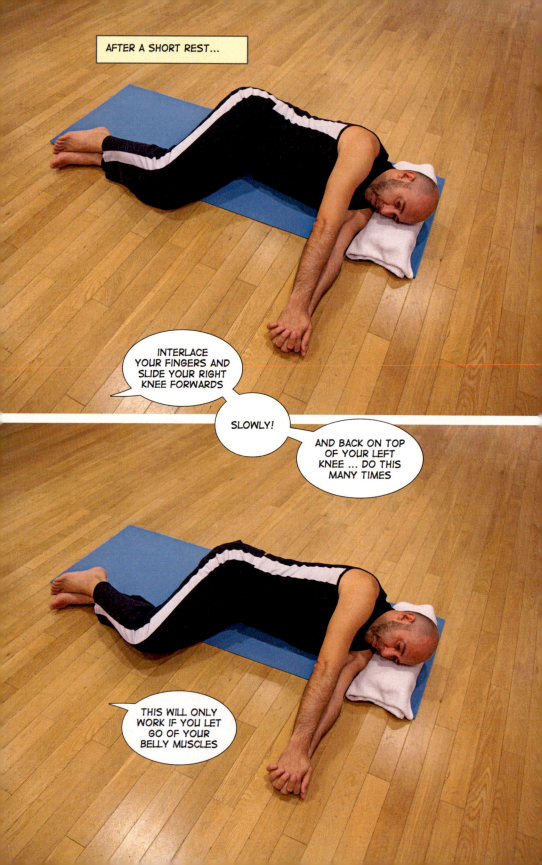

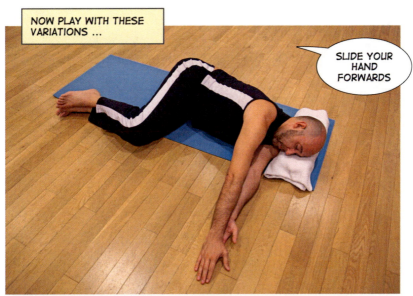

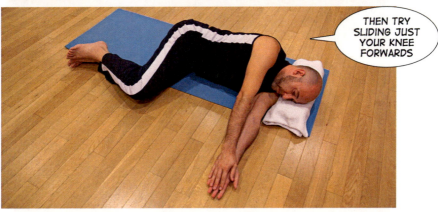

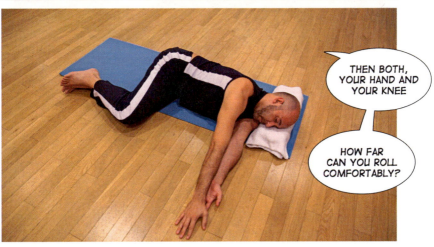

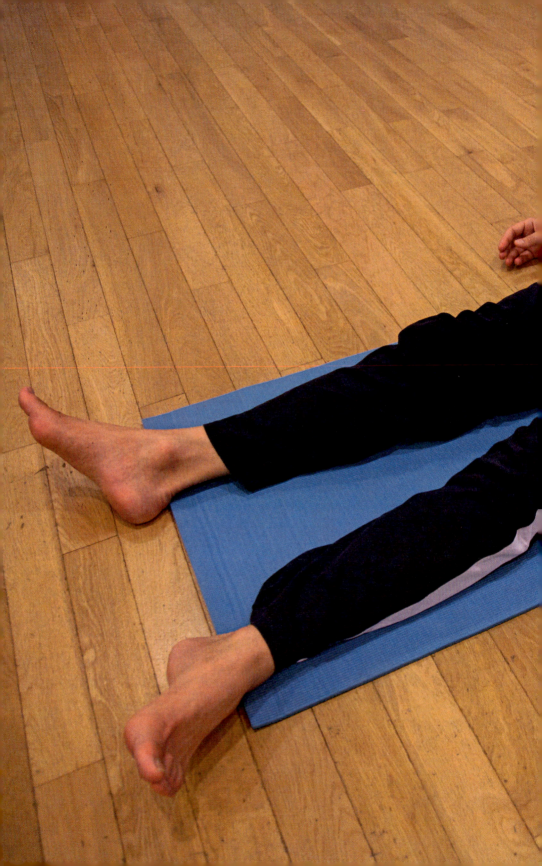

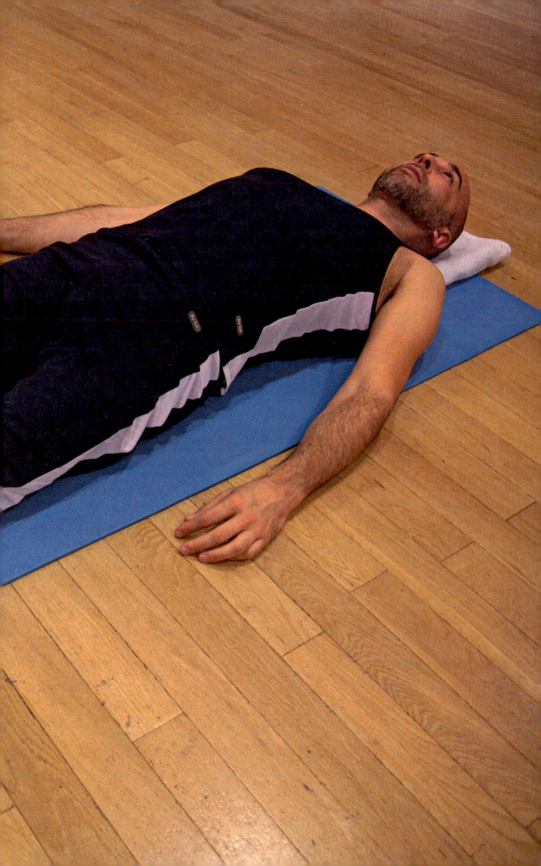

There is a difference in how he rests his left leg on the floor, as opposed to his right leg; this can be observed about his hands and arms too. However, we don't ask if this is correct or not. Maybe his head is turned a tiny bit more to his left, even though the neck is relaxed. In real life you could also observe his chest being moved by his breathing. Is his breathing more evenly, solemnly, equitably distributed over his whole chest, his whole self, compared to before the lesson?

As you can see it's a nice sensation to just lie on the floor and be perfectly comfortable; maybe to be aware of gravity, of where there is contact with the floor, of the breath, friendly sensations coming in from the neck and shoulders. After a Feldenkrais lesson, there is a particular sense of inner peace and being aware of one self.

Play with movement initiation

Most everything starts somewhere. For movement, a signal is sent to some muscles: these are the muscles that will be contracted first, and thus start to make something move. Other muscles will jump in later; but it certainly starts somewhere. Where does it start?

The start will determine how the action will be going, how the body organizes itself according to the intended move, and how good the actual move will be. The skill here is to focus on where a movement starts and to organize movements from there on, using various starting points. With different starting points, there will be differences in body organization and differences in the efficiency and quality of a movement. You must be able to feel what's happening inside yourself in order to play with movement initiation. Plus you may make conscious choices of what movement-quality you want — e. g. powerful, fast, slow, investigative, gentle…

But what does it mean to have different starting points? Take turning the head, for example: you can focus on your entire head turning. But you can also just focus on the tip of your nose, or on your ear, or on your cheek. You could bring your attention to the eyes first, and then let them lead the rest of yourself. Or you could focus on the tip of your nose and the back of your head at the same time (if the nose turns to the left, the back of the head will turn to the right). Focusing on more than one spot will increase the difficulty of the exploration, but also increase your skillz.

To quote Moshé Feldenkrais: „The point is that there is nothing, nothing that we do not learn – in its breadth and understanding since childhood – even the simplest movements. That is why there are very strange things. For instance, if someone says »Do a movement with the head up and down«, when the person makes one movement up, you can see that when the person thinks of the movement up and down – he only thinks of the nose. The nose does the movement up and down. If you tell him to think that he is doing the movement down with a point behind his head, it seems strange to him. You will see that there is an enormous difference. The one, who does it with his nose, moves like this and the one, who does it with the point behind the head, does it like that. That is why you see such different and varied movements between two people."

Another practical example, from Adrienne Glazov, Feldenkrais Practitioner. She reports: „In my first lesson I most often teach movement initiation. People find it fascinating how many different places that one movement can be initiated." She then continues with a story about practicing her own teachings during a skiing holiday: „I was skiing and I did not like my turns. It seemed like my left ankle was stiff. How to get it to ease up? I practice what I teach. First, I started 'drawing' my turn with my arm. I found it wasn't only my ankle, it was my ribs that were not turning. A little further, I found I didn't need such a large arc, and my concentration turned to the fact that my toes on my left foot were curled. I focused on the spot between my big toe and the second toe and made sure that the spot touched down. Pretty soon, the tension released and I got it all together. That was a gift for the day."

Usually you will have habitual ways of doing things. And sometimes, when you feel stuck, the more effort you put forth, the more you will have the feeling of being stuck. One of the things you can learn to do in Feldenkrais classes, like in Adrienne's skiing example, is initiating movement from different places. You will find that you can actually choose from many possibilities, and that you can improve casually and adapt to demanding situations more easily.

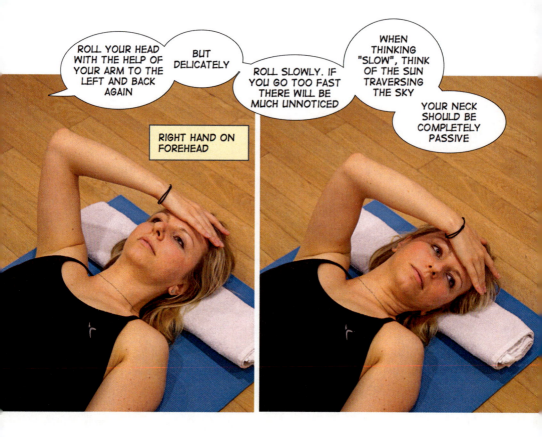

Rolling the head

This is a short part of a longer lesson. I include this „snippet" to illustrate the learning process of how to reduce muscular effort, find pathways, and vary movement initiation; it's always nice to study by using a real life example. In addition to this, it's another great little exercise for reducing tension in the neck.

The lesson starts in supine position, lying on the back. To guide students into this lesson, it might be helpful to give a few cues: „feel the floor behind your head. It's just there. Reliably so. Your head is resting on it. Your head is supported by it. No need to hold your head. No need to hold your shoulders. They are carried by the floor. Feel the weight of your head weighing on the pillow. Let go, let your head and shoulders rest."

Then we're all set to engage into the business of rolling the head, just like in the picture story. There's a couple of challenges in this short lesson: being able to do it slowly, and being able to alternate between us-

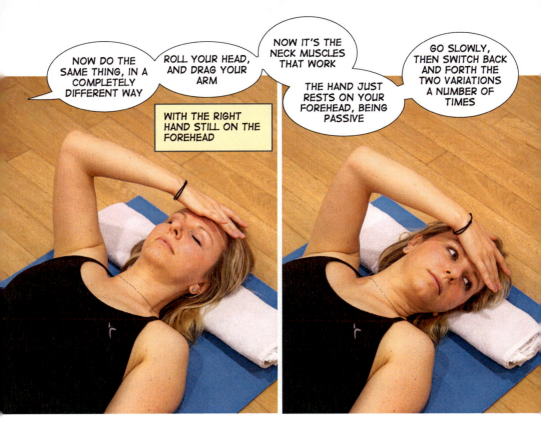

ing the arm to roll the head, and using the neck muscles to roll the head. And to be able to sense minimal differences. Being able to move delicately and to sense minimal differences go hand in hand.

Every person will experience this kind of rolling slightly differently. For example, there will be differences in trajectory (is the head rolling more in a curve or more in a straight line?), in the smoothness of movement (is it a bit jerky, with stops in between?), in how much the shoulder girdle and chest are participating, in the movements of the eyes, and how much the eyes support or impede rolling... and a lot more.

There's a reason for all those differences: it's a complicated matter! Let's review what the neck is comprised of: there's not only 7 vertebrae (plus 12 in the chest) but also about 29 groups of muscles in the neck, some of them spanning as little as two vertebrae at a time. All these muscles need to be coordinated and directed and inhibited by the nervous system. And there's ribs and a sternum and clavicles and many ligaments and tendons, and reflexes, and habits and a human being, with a life and movement habits, experience and a personal history.

Knowledge and knowing

A scholar consulted a sage as to
how separate parts create a whole
and what differentiates knowledge of the many
from knowledge of the whole.
The sage answered:
What is widely dispersed becomes an entity only
when it finds its centre.
For what is myriad
achieves substance and significance
only at the centre
and then its abundance looks like simplicity —
almost like nothing
a fruitful void, a calm force
gravitating towards
that which gives it meaning.

To experience the whole
or share in it
we do not need to know every detail,
neither do we need to speak of everything
nor have or do all.
To enter into the heart of the city
we only have to walk through one gate.
Many tones reverberate
in the striking of a single bell.
And when we pick a ripe apple
we need not know how it came to be as it is.
We take it in our hands and eat it.

The scholar argued with
the sage: to grasp the truth,
we must first know all the facts.
But the sage contradicted him:
only when the truth is grown old
can we begin to know all the facts.
Truth which makes us move on
is risky
and untried.

This truth conceals its promise
as the seed conceals the tree within.
Therefore if we hesitate to act because
we want to know more
than we need for our next step,
we miss the chance to grow.
We accept small change in place of riches
and out of living trees make firewood.

The scholar immediately remarked
that this was surely only part of the answer,
and begged the wise man for some more.
The wise man waved aside this question,
knowing that fullness resembles a barrel of fresh cider
– sweet and cloudy.
It needs fermentation and sufficient time
until it clears.
If instead of savouring it, we try to gulp it down
we become befuddled and unsteady.

from the book „Insights: Lectures and Stories" by Bert Hellinger.
Permission to reprint courtesy of Bert Hellinger.

The journey is the reward

We need to get things done – and often we don't care (aka don't have time) for the details along the way. Then most everything is goal oriented, and the body serves to achieve these goals. There is an seemingly endless number of things to do, aka goals to reach, in daily life, work, sports, recreation, and so on.

Our lives revolve around reaching goals, accomplishing tasks: thousands and thousands each day. Therefore, there is no time to focus on the movements themselves — or is there?
We probably won't get anything done if we tried to explore and figure out every movement anew every time. Accomplishing things is done by intent and habits. Habits govern movements. But in order to improve movement, one must be able to observe movement itself. While going for a goal, one must learn to bring attention to the movement and how it is executed.

Bringing attention to the movement itself, as opposed to solely focusing on a goal, will reveal *how* things are done. Besides the solid, practical aspects, there are also emotional and spiritual ones: the Taoists say, „The Journey is the reward", and they built a whole philosophy on it. You may also have seen this famous saying anywhere from self-help books to car sales ads.

More poetically, Paulo Coelho writes: „A warrior of light practices a powerful exercise for inner growth: he pays attention to the things he does automatically, such as breathing, blinking, or noticing the things around him. [..] In this way he frees himself from tensions and allows his intuition to work more freely, without interference from his fears and desires. Certain problems that appeared to be insoluble are resolved, certain sorrows from which he thought he would never recover vanish naturally."

It doesn't take much effort to learn to focus on the present moment and on your actual moves, nor is it difficult. However, it's not something that you will master in one lesson. It needs a bit of commitment, persistence and attentive study. In this way, the successful journey will be quite casual. While there may be a plenitude of philosophical aspects, in

Feldenkrais classes we focus on learning in a practical sense. What you do with it and however else you take advantage of it is entirely up to you.

Employ your muscles to their best purpose

Every muscle (or group of muscles) is good for some functions, and not as good for other functions. For example, the Biceps brachii are best at „supination" of the forearm (turning the palm upwards), not at flexion of the elbow, as one may expect. For a layman it might come as a surprise that the most powerful muscle for flexing the elbow is the deeper-lying Brachialis muscle. However, the Biceps can help with flexion. Furthermore, both Brachialis and Biceps, can assist other muscles with forward flexion of the shoulder joint (bringing the arm forward and upwards), horizontal adduction (bringing the arm across the body) and a couple other moves.

The important point here is not Latin names and abstract concepts of which muscles are good for doing what — but to be aware that muscles can support each other as well as work against each other. And that certain muscles can be over- and underused.

When a muscle is used for a movement that it's not meant to do normally, or if it's disturbing other muscles' work, in Feldenkrais we call this „parasitic action". We use this strong term because instead of contributing, these muscles draw energy from a movement and make it less efficient, maybe even painful in the long run. In other modalities this is called „energy leak". I guess Dr. Moshé Feldenkrais coined it „parasitic" because he was a scientist, and had parasitic battery drains in mind.

So instead of merely going for anatomy books and studying which muscle is supposed to do what in theory, we study movements and functional relationships for real with Feldenkrais lessons. And then go back to the books (maybe). It's like finding an interesting specimen on a walk. It raises curiosity naturally. In this way, we don't just study anatomy intellectually, but with the body and mind and all the senses at the same time.

Trust in self-organization

In one lesson Moshé Feldenkrais gave the following advice: „Do it more gently at the points where it is difficult. Do not try to push more, but at the points where it is difficult, do it more easily, a gentler movement, more slowly. Then, slowly it will organize itself." He does not say, „then, you will be able to organize it" or „then you will know how to do it".

The key phrase here is „then it will organize itself". It is the nervous system that organizes movement. And a healthy nervous system will always try to make the best possible choice, given the information and possibilities available at the time.

Let's look at another example, this time from blogger Jeff Sexton. He writes about his swimming skills and how he improved his backstroke: „I was a lousy backstroker, with a flaccid flutter kick and stiff shoulders that weren't double-jointed like most talented backstrokers' were. But my turning point from awful to good arrived with this bit of wisdom from Coach Emery: »Don't worry about putting your pinkie in the water first; that's bad advice. Just relax your arm and roll your body as you swing your arm back into the water. Your pinky will naturally enter the water first – without you worrying about it – and you'll have better mechanics.« Once I started focusing on the principles behind the mechanics – and not on the outer form of the mechanics – my entire stroke transformed."

Jeff demonstrates the same lesson: our movements can be rather complex, and focusing on the details and how to do things „right" can quickly add up to be more trouble than help. In this way, we don't focus on how to get our movements right, but trust that the nervous system, provide with enough choices, will eventually figure it out.

Another example is how to breathe the „right way"; although the heated discussion between health professionals has calmed down a bit in the last couple of centuries, contrary viewpoints still remain and may never be resolved. Other debates include: how to hold the pelvis the right way – what is the correct degree of anterior tilt? And how to walk and run and where to place the feet when running; is it the heels or the balls of the feet – or somewhere in between?

Such questions are difficult to answer and every couple of years there is a new expert with an even better solution. The obvious, as well as the subtle, ingredients for every posture and action are so many that we can't control them all. It's impossible. And there's no joy in doing so either.

Therefore, learning to trust in ones' central nervous system and its ability to organize itself during Feldenkrais classes (or e. g. during times of coaching, like in the backstroke example), is by far the smartest, safest and most pleasant way to find the most suitable movements for a given situation.

Look beyond habits

In Feldenkrais group classes students are guided through movement sequences, exploring each move several times, usually between two and twenty times. Movements are done in a way that supports exploration and the gathering of knowledge about oneself. Students are moving and observing at the same time.

If there are no habits governing a certain move, learning is possible right away. For example, a rather difficult and unusual instruction would be: „first open your mouth a bit, then shift your chin to the left while sticking your tongue to the right". Since (for most people) there is no established habit and little knowledge about this movement, it's easy to jump right into exploring how to do it.

For very common tasks we do many hundred times per day, like turning the head to the left and back to centre again, everyone has their way of doing so. It's far more difficult to look at the details of this move because they are hidden by habits. To look beyond these habits and become aware of the actual movement, is a key learning requisite in the Feldenkrais Method. Being able to learn to focus on movement itself (instead of focusing on a goal) is an intrinsic part of every lesson.

To access a movement like turning the head, we would, for example, lie supine, and have the head rest on the floor or a pillow. In this way it's easier to observe subtle sensations than in an upright position. Then we could go into, just for example, differentiating eye and head movements („roll the head to the left, while looking to the right").

Once „control-by-habit" has been overruled, movement lies open to be observed. Particular details will become apparent. The movement will be jerky at some places, smoother at others; faster at some, slower at others. At some points a movement will feel comfortable, some will feel unsatisfactory. Sometimes a movement will bring up feelings; sometimes it will feel dull or inaccessible. There are so many things to experience. All that is usually hidden by habits.

Resolving the red light reflex

Thomas Hanna (1928-1990), President of the Humanistic Psychology Institute (HPI), Feldenkrais practitioner, Organizer of the first Feldenkrais Professional Training in San Francisco 1975, founder of Hanna Somatic Education®, invented the term „somatics". In his book „Somatics: Reawakening the Mind's Control of Movement, Flexibility, and Health" he gives a solution to a problem that was thoroughly defined by Hans Selye.

„Who was Hans Selye" you might ask? In case you never heard of him, a super brief introduction too: Hans Selye (1907–1982), born in Vienna, Austria, was a pioneering endocrinologist. He became a Doctor of Medicine and Chemistry in Prague, Czech Rebublic, and spent most of his life in Montréal, Canada. During his life time he earned 43 (!) titles of honorary doctor, authored over 1,000 research publications, 15 monographs and 7 popular books. Just like Thomas Hanna, he as well created a new term, a term so popular that everyone is using it: „stressed".

Thomas Hanna identified three reflexive postural tendencies caused by stress, and coined one of them „the red light reflex". He explains that this involuntary reflex pattern contracts all the muscles of the front side of the body. It is triggered by negative feelings such as fear, worry, apprehension, and sadness. Signs of this habituated pattern include rounded shoulders, the head extended forward over the body, sore neck and shoulder muscles, contracted abdominal muscles, shallow breathing, depression, digestion problems, constipation, and many more. In this regard, Thomas Hanna writes: „By learning to regain both awareness, sensation, and motor control of muscles – an educational process that can only be achieved through movement – the brain can remember how to relax and move the muscles properly."

To start to resolve this „red light reflex", just for example, we use the following Feldenkrais movement sequence. You will find this sequence in Thomas Hanna's book, as well as in most courses or books teaching Feldenkrais lessons. Even in this one. Let's see how it's done:

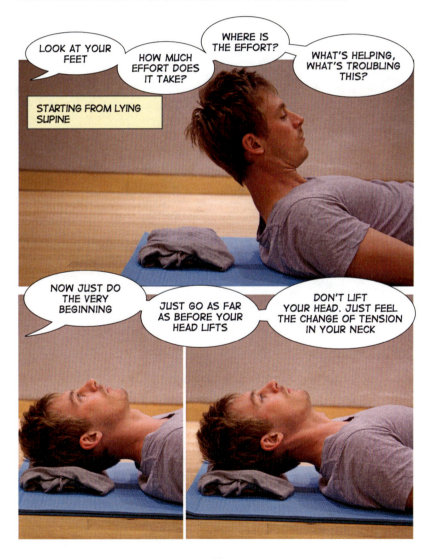

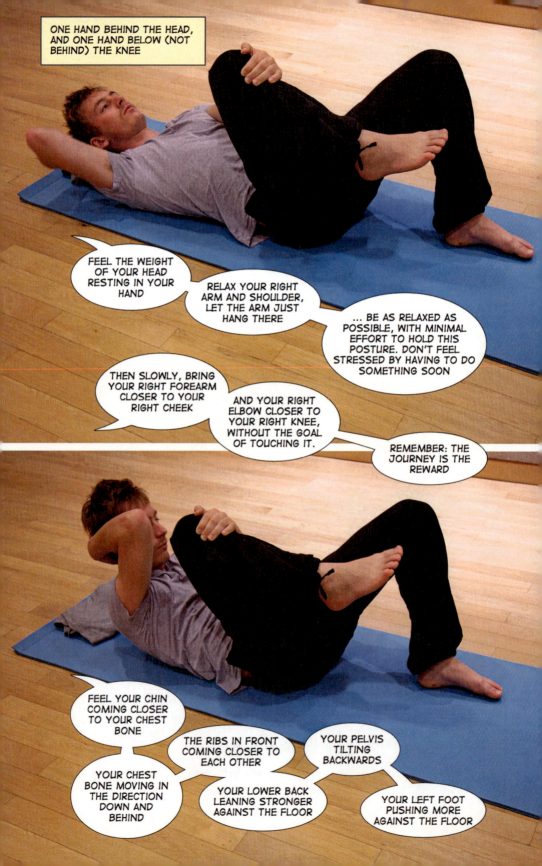

It can't be stressed (here it is again) enough, that this should be done in a relaxed fashion. By the way, why do we use forward flexion to release tension patterns that cause forward flexion and contraction of the flexor muscles on the front side? Because in this manner we can get aware of the tension, and the nervous system can finally register and let go. This is a very important strategy used often in Feldenkrais classes. Feldenkrais practitioners call it „to go with the pattern".

Frequent, short pauses in lying supine in Feldenkrais classes are not to recover from exhaustion. Actually there are several types of such pauses. One is to observe things (e. g. the contact with the floor or the tension in the neck) and check what has changed, one is to let the breathing calm down (if it was disturbed or agitated), one is to a take a break to be able to make a fresh start. Any other reasons?

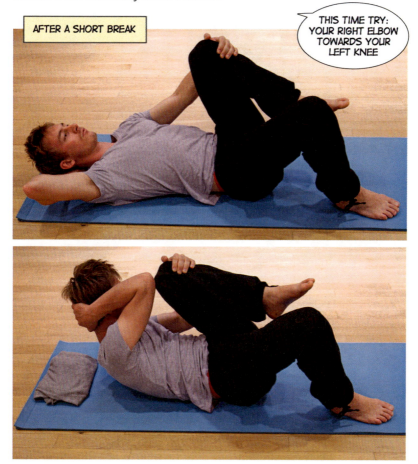

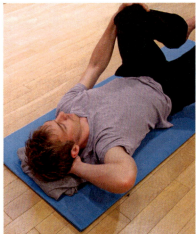 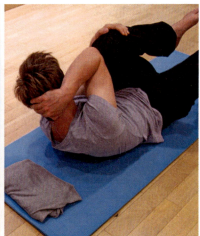

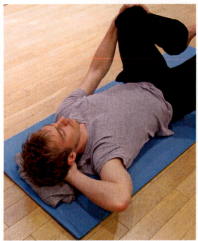 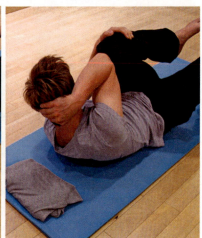

RATHER THAN REPEATING THE SAME MOVE OVER AND OVER, LOOK FOR VARIATIONS AND POSSIBILITIES WITH EACH REPETITION. YOU CAN SEE GULLIAUME IS AIMING AT A DIFFERENT SPOT ON HIS KNEE, EVERY TIME HE CURLS UP GENTLY. YOU WILL NOTICE: ONE TIME IT'S MORE OF A TWIST, THE OTHER IT'S MORE OF A STRAIGHT FORWARD FLEXION.

AND ONCE EVERY SO OFTEN TRY TO LET YOUR ELBOW SINK BACK TO THE FLOOR – IN ORDER TO BE ABLE TO START YOUR NEXT MOVEMENT JUST AS IT WAS YOUR FIRST.

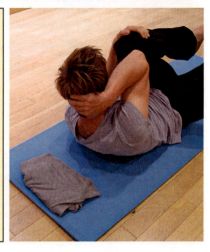

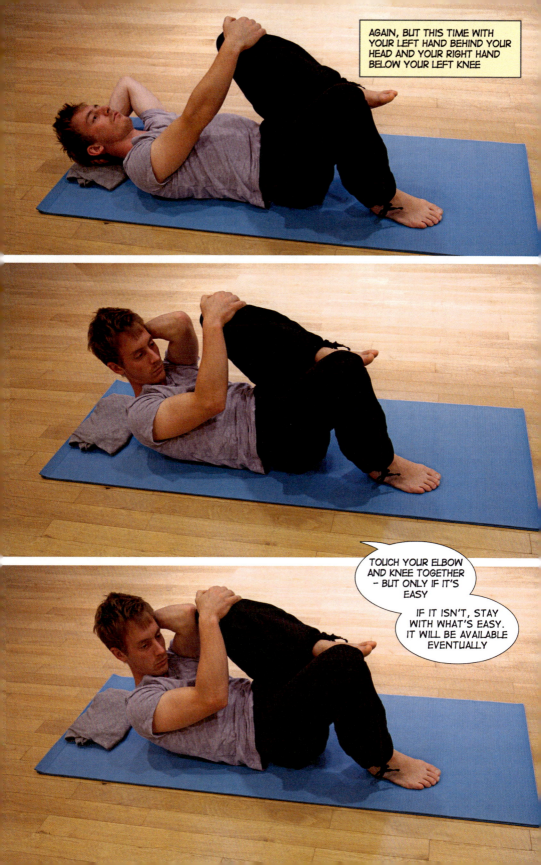

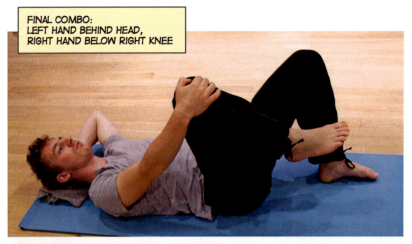

FINAL COMBO:
LEFT HAND BEHIND HEAD,
RIGHT HAND BELOW RIGHT KNEE

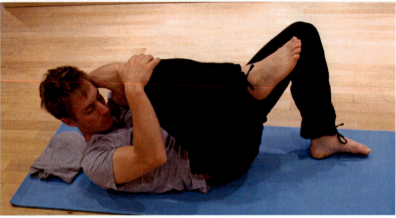

Even if done slowly and attentively, it's impossible to catch all the benefits in one go. The more often a lesson is done, the more one can discover. However, because repetition can hide details and dull interest, there are many other lessons similar to this one. One can do various lessons, and at a later point return to a specific one. It will be different. It's like rediscovering one's favourite book after it sat on the shelf for a couple of years.

To round up this lesson hold your head in your hands again, gently bring elbows and knees into proximity, then just hang in there, breath, relax, enjoy. You could slowly, slightly roll from one side to the other, feel how your weight is shifted from left to right, the weight of your limbs, organs; even your brain, that is nicely floating inside your skull. Or you could bring your feet slightly closer to the floor, keeping the distance between elbows and knees, and roll back and forth like this. You will find joy in these little things.

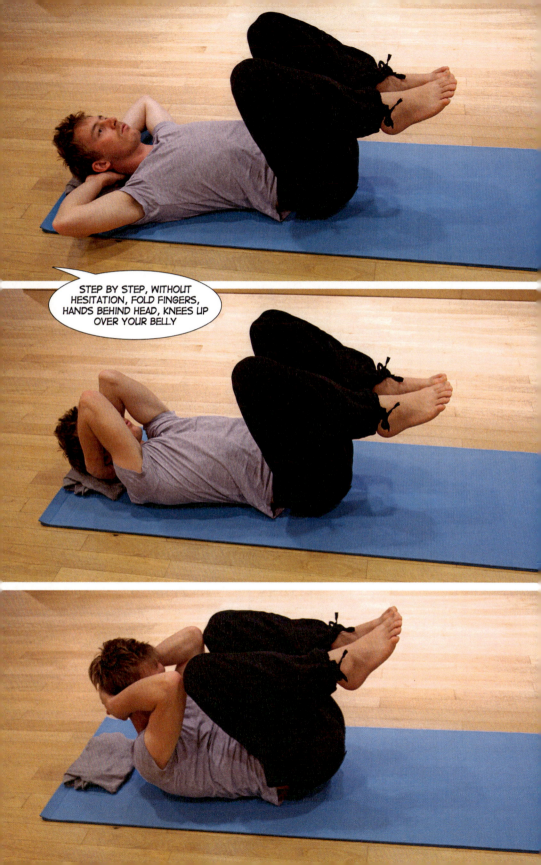

Resolving the green light reflex

Some lessons really fit together quite well. For example forward flexion goes nicely together with backward extension. They do not only complement each other, but if done one after the other, or taking turns even, they form a synergy and enhance each other.

The green light reflex (as coined by Thomas Hanna) involuntary contracts all the muscles of the back of the body. It might also be addressed as „positive stress" or „eustress". This kind of stress can give an extra burst of adrenaline to help you accomplish goals and meet deadlines. Eustress provides mental alertness, motivation, and efficiency. However, if the muscles of the back of the body are triggered often enough, and rarely relaxed deliberately, they might just keep being contracted. It is said that signs of this pattern include low back pain, neck stiffness, tight shoulder muscles, and tight hamstrings. Over time, this wear and tear might cause physical damage to the spine, in form of delaminated layers or circumferential rents in the discs, damaged vertebrae and vertebral endplates, or even disc herniation. In Feldenkrais we view this as a functional problem that requires relearning, rather than just stretching, adjustment, gym workout to strengthen the muscles, or massage.

In this regard Prof. Dr. Stuart McGill, professor for spine biomechanics at the University of Waterloo, Canada, writes: „Many clinicians follow a recipe for assessment, treatment or performance training. Using this generic approach ensures average results – some patients/clients will improve and get better, but many will fail. The first step in any exercise progression is to remove the cause of the pain, namely the perturbed motion and motor patterns [..] This need not be so complicated. The clinician addresses the postural cause and corrects standing to shut the muscles off and remove the associated crushing load from the spine. The client exclaims: You're magical – you just took the ache out of my back!" And that's exactly what we try to do here, in a Feldenkrais sort of way.

To know what this lesson feels like, it's crucial to do it yourself, preferably with guidance of a Feldenkrais Practitioner. The Practitioner will teach it in a way in which you will have a learning situation, find study points, and have an overall pleasurable, beneficial experience.

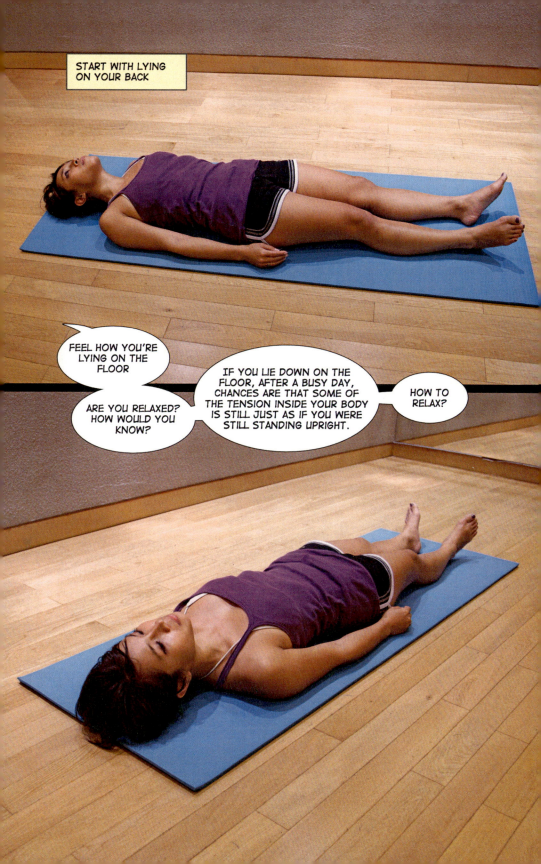

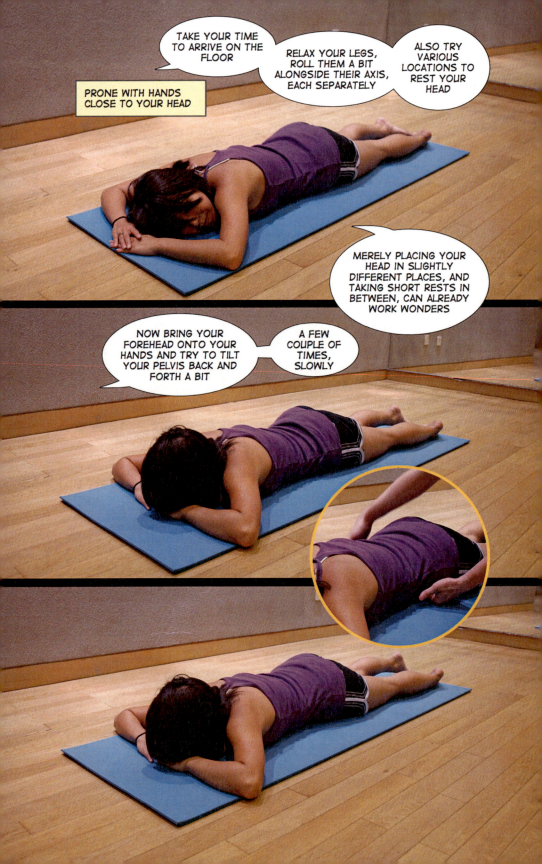

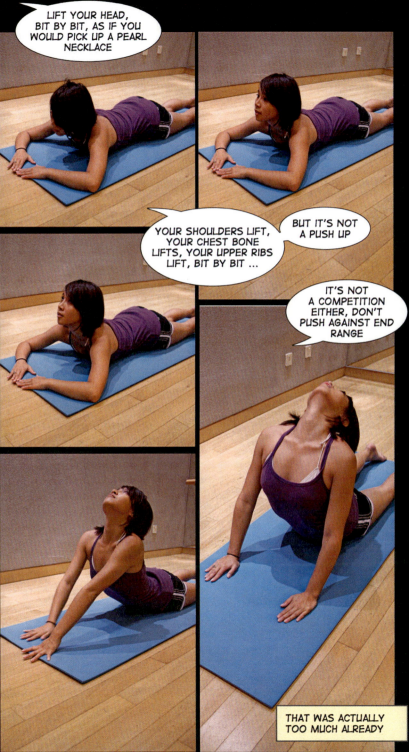

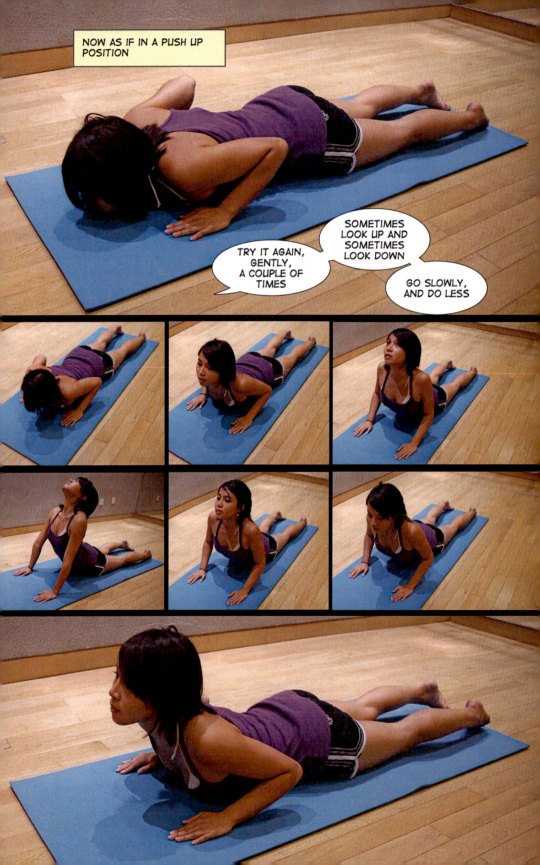

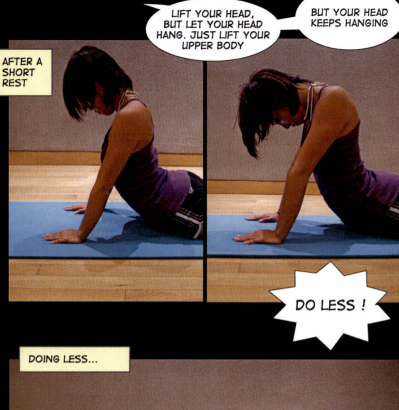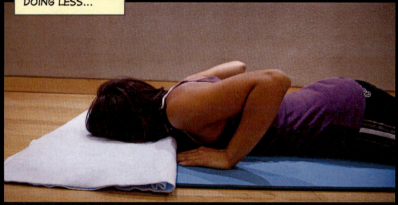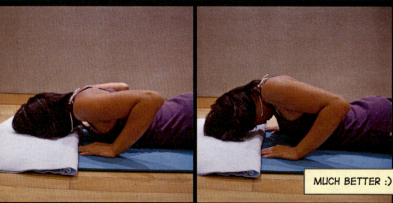

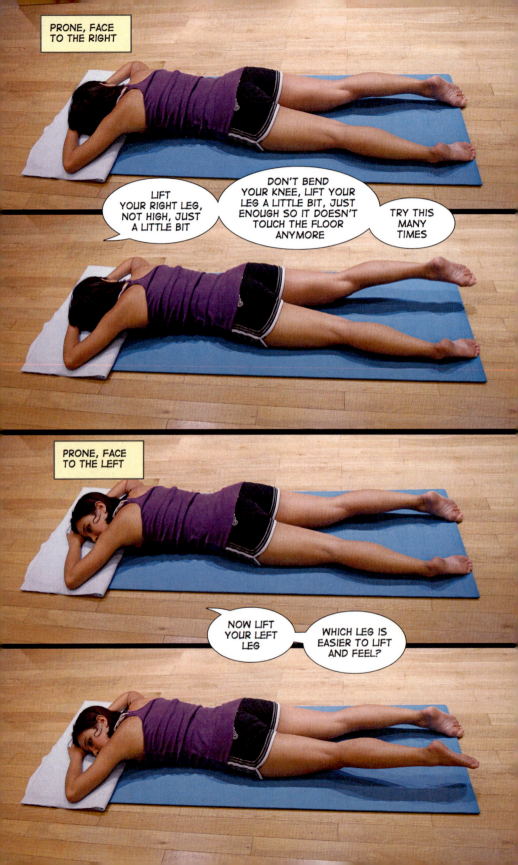

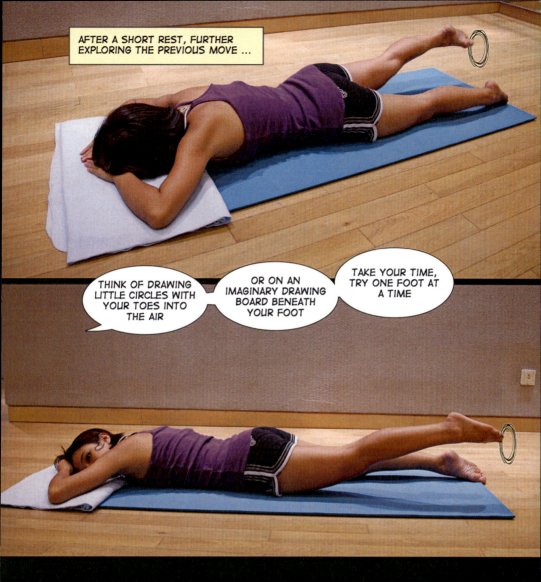

Drawing circles can be introduced gradually, by breaking the movement down into some of its components: up and down, as well as left and right. Try to draw smooth lines first. Then, the far ends of the lines can be connected, quarter by quarter, to eventually form a full circle.

Bring awareness to a number of points: is it a circle or more of a square or polygon? Are the toes pointing straight or is the ankle bent? Where are you leaning against, your pubic bone, iliac crest, belly, chest? Are both directions, clockwise and counterclockwise, of equal smoothness and speed, without jerks? These questions make this movement interesting. Merely focusing on the task of lifting the leg and doing circles would be quite a boring exercise, instead of a learning situation.

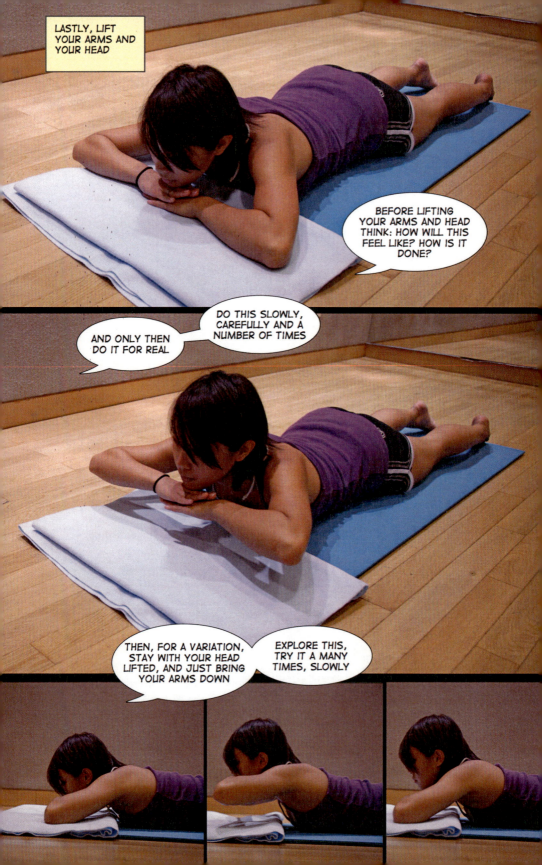

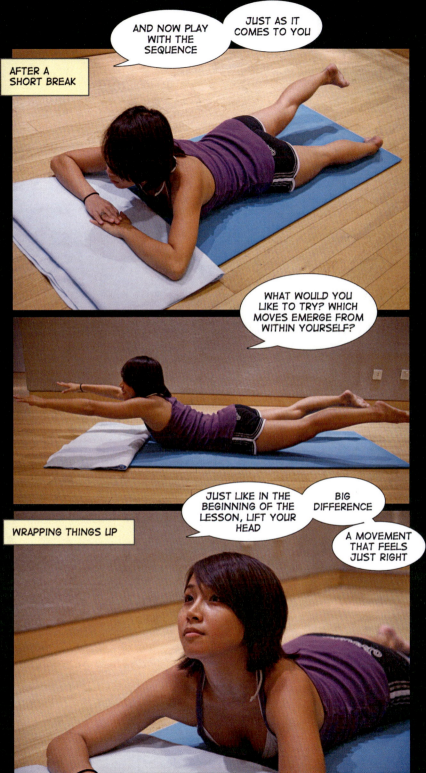

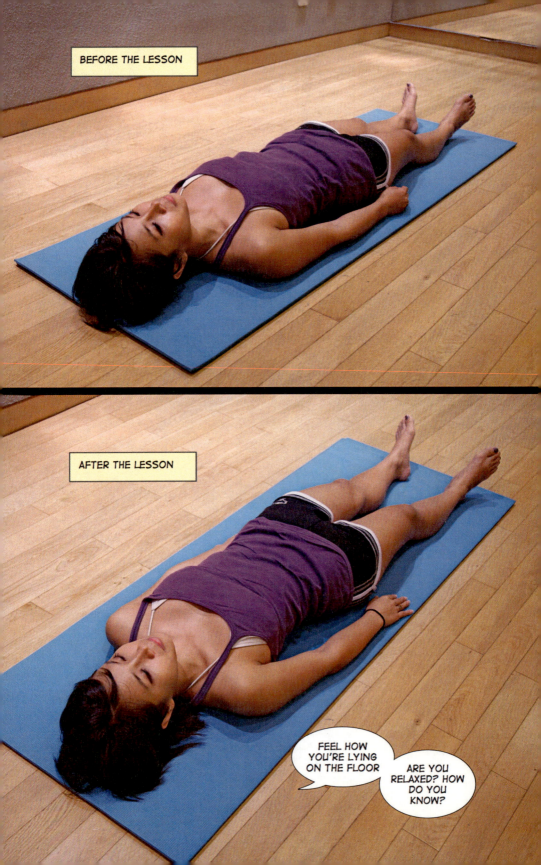

Find what's interesting

Not all of what we have to do is interesting, not all is pleasurable; among our duties we may have some things we don't want to do at all. The same goes for our body movements; not all movements are interesting and maybe some are even painful or not pleasurable at all. Usually these will be blanked out and submitted to habits (or other automatisms).

In the worst cases, not only single movements, but also whole passages of a day can be „lost" this way... like driving to work, or eating lunch in the same restaurant with the same people over and over again. However, in life one can always find parts that are interesting and worth taking a look at. It's simply a question of how to find them.

In every Feldenkrais lesson there is a main theme and maybe secondary themes supporting the main theme. For the main theme, a continued novelty needs to be maintained throughout the lesson. Once the novelty wears off, awareness is dulled and learning no longer takes place. Therefore new situations and movements are presented.

The key here is to find something interesting in a physical movement. To find something that catches one's attention for a while. For sure there is something. Feldenkrais lessons are made for students to discover something. Maybe think of a visit to an art gallery and having to find something interesting in a painting. There certainly is some detail or related story to discover. Btw, „Interesse" is Latin and means „to differ, to be important".

Joy through simplicity

People seek feelings in extremes. The golfer sets out on the course to find this certain „ping" where he hits the ball just right. A single fraction of a second can make his day. The skier looks for the perfect swing, while indulging in the perfect conditions – blue sky, crisp air, stunning views. He doesn't mind the effort and cost, if he only gets that high feeling. The modern yoga student tries to go into unusual postures to find satisfaction in the extraordinary. The classic yoga students sits for hours without movement and an empty mind. The motorcyclist gets his rush by opening the valves, going into tunnel vision, adrenaline pumping into his bloodstream. He risks his life just to get a feeling of being present.

A big misconception about movement is that one can only find deep appreciation and joy of being in the present moment trough extreme situations; that it doesn't last long, and that it doesn't happen often; maybe even that you have to pay for it.

Therefore, it might come as good news that ordinary movement can provide the same kind of feelings, without the use of drugs, without meditation techniques, without strenuous efforts or high costs. These feelings of joy for ordinary movement are available on request, in every breath, in each simple move.

Discovering the joy of simple movements and the delightful relationship between moving and thinking is part of Feldenkrais classes. Again and again this kind of discovery can be seen in classes. People release unnecessary tension and expectations for great things to happen, and start to feel and appreciate themselves.

It's not just what students say after class, but such changes can be seen in class, when the gaze turns inwards, breathing becomes rhythmical, not interfered by movements, thoughts, or speech, and the expressions on the faces appear calm and content. Being able to enjoy movement is not just therapeutic but natural.

Explore real movements

Diets, fitness exercises, workout programs: what was right three years ago might be considered obsolete today — maybe even harmful. This happens again and again.

Nevertheless, most therapists and personal trainers aren't afraid to tell you what to do; they will tell you the right way to sit, to run, to lift, to breathe, to live your life. They'll tell you what to eat, how much to drink, and how many sheets it takes to wipe. The more popular ones will do so without even looking at you. What all those authorities have in common is that they impose knowledge — may it be from personal experience or from academic study — onto you, the client.

In Feldenkrais classes, students are invited to quite a different way. Instead of trying to tell them how to move correctly, e. g. getting up from sitting to standing correctly, or sitting correctly, standing correctly, walking correctly, to turn correctly (and so forth), students shall develop the feel of what's actually happening when they engage in a movement.

First and foremost this is about bringing attention to specific movements. For example, how a certain joint moves naturally, and how it moves in relation to the rest of the body. This can be as simple as the first (and second and third) joint in your pointer finger on your dominant hand. In which directions does it flex/extend easiest? From anatomy books we know it's a hinge joint. An anatomy book may say: „A hinge joint allows extension and retraction of an appendage [..]" Such definitions are very precise, but also quite abstract – even with a nicely drawn, detailed picture. Some anatomy books go into great detail, with fascinating pictures from carefully chosen angles.

Yet how is this intellectual knowledge transferred into the body? This is quite a significant question – and the answer cannot be found within the realm of mind and reason. It's not enough to just memorize anatomy books. A quick wiggle of a particular joint won't make a memorable, beneficial experience either. To make the transition from intellect to physical reality, one has to engage in a learning experience that includes the body as well as the mind.

Continuing with the example, the first (or second) joint on the index finger is not the same in every person. In fact, every person's finger joints work a little bit differently.

You can see some people are able to stretch and flex their fingers more than others, and for some the fingers are not straight but curved to one or the other side. For some the movement feels easy and flexible; for others it feels stiff and unhappy. It's different for everyone, and different over the years. Does it flex easiest in a straight line? Or is it easiest with a bit of a rotation? Does it extend as easy as it flexes? Is slow and small as available as fast and strong? And when you let go, where is the rest position? Is the rest position after having extended the finger the same as after having it flexed? (It's not). It really is an exploration of real movements. Discover and develop a feel for how you really move around, and not just how you should, according to what other people say.

The flexible spine

The human spine is a marvellous structure that does it all: flexion, extension, rotation. It can be stiff and can bear loads that try to compress, shear and twist it, yet it can be supple and flexible and allow movement in many kinds of patterns and directions.

The following is a rather tricky lesson, which is composed of many parts. Each part could indeed be a full lesson on its on, each page broken up into 10 or more pages. From afar it looks like as if the previous two lessons are intertwined, and the result is a strong flexion and extension performed by the spine at the same time.

Furthermore, this lesson is an inversion: the head is in a position lower than the heart. In the Yoga community inversions are praised for its many health benefits, and to quote Yoga Journal: „Headstand and Shoulderstand are known as the king and queen of the asanas".

A word of caution though: if you suffer from low back pain I recommend to stay far away from this lesson (and any gymnastic exercises that are similar, such as supine leg lifts). Swinging the legs up imposes considerable loads and forces on the lower back. Instead of indulging into difficult exercises, injury avoidance is a safe bet on the way to recovery. In order to do this lesson safely, proper core strength, contraction-relaxation speed, and coordination is required; as well as an uninjured lower back, which can successfully bear load.

Finding this kind of organisation, coordination and movement is not trivial. It's perfectly ok to take your time. If a smooth flow can't be discovered during a class, maybe it will sometime at home, or in the next weeks or even months. There's no hurry.

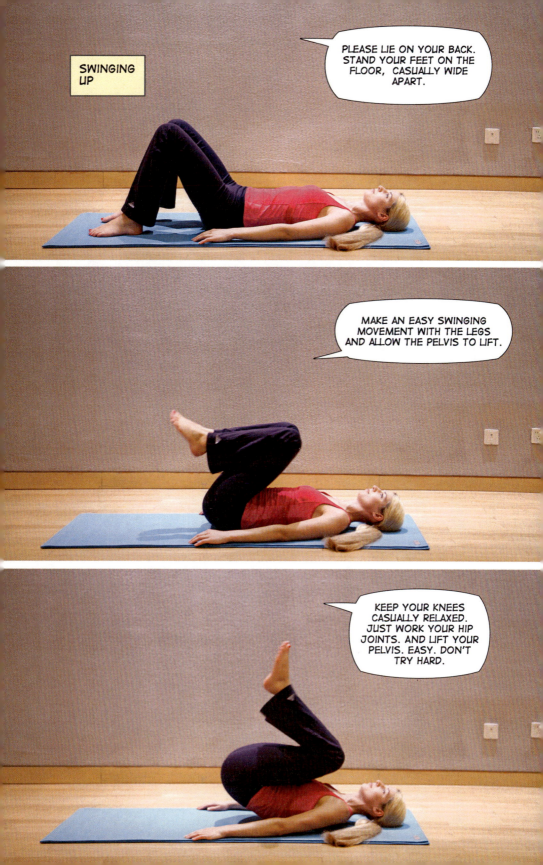

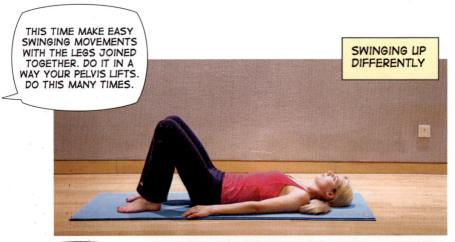

SWINGING UP DIFFERENTLY

"THIS TIME MAKE EASY SWINGING MOVEMENTS WITH THE LEGS JOINED TOGETHER. DO IT IN A WAY YOUR PELVIS LIFTS. DO THIS MANY TIMES."

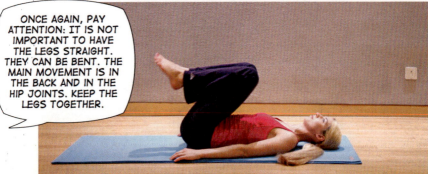

"ONCE AGAIN, PAY ATTENTION: IT IS NOT IMPORTANT TO HAVE THE LEGS STRAIGHT. THEY CAN BE BENT. THE MAIN MOVEMENT IS IN THE BACK AND IN THE HIP JOINTS. KEEP THE LEGS TOGETHER."

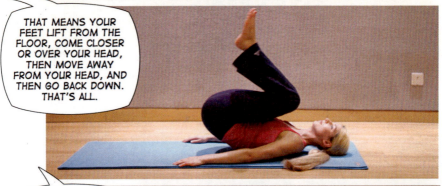

"THAT MEANS YOUR FEET LIFT FROM THE FLOOR, COME CLOSER OR OVER YOUR HEAD, THEN MOVE AWAY FROM YOUR HEAD, AND THEN GO BACK DOWN. THAT'S ALL."

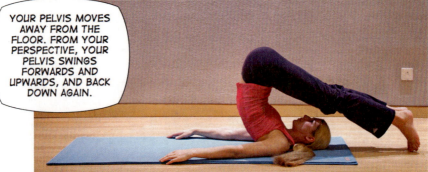

"YOUR PELVIS MOVES AWAY FROM THE FLOOR. FROM YOUR PERSPECTIVE, YOUR PELVIS SWINGS FORWARDS AND UPWARDS, AND BACK DOWN AGAIN."

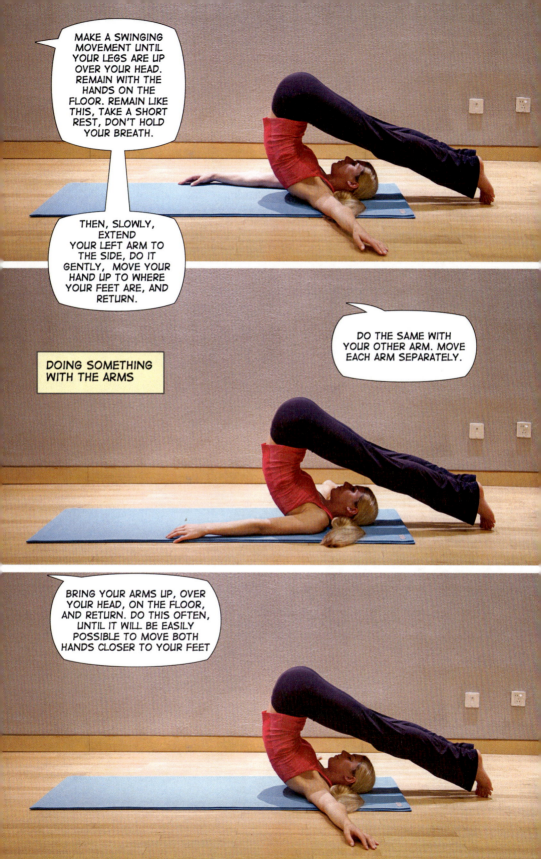

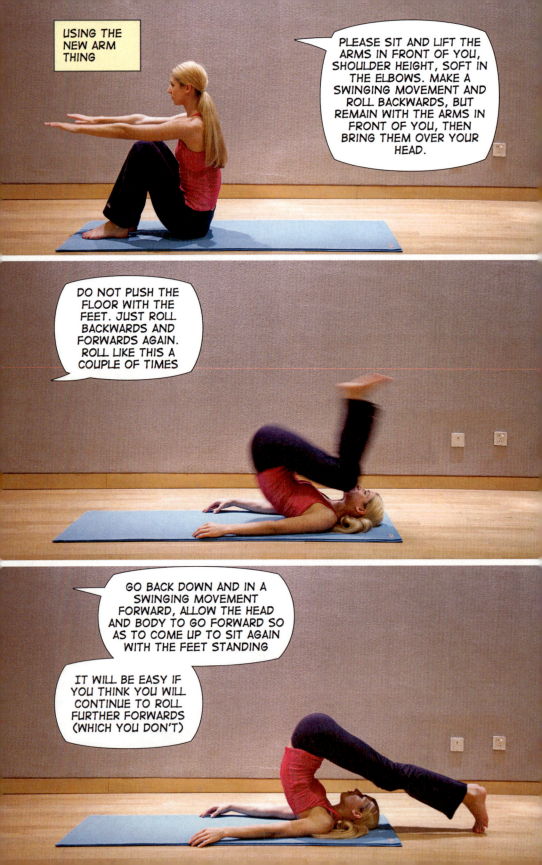

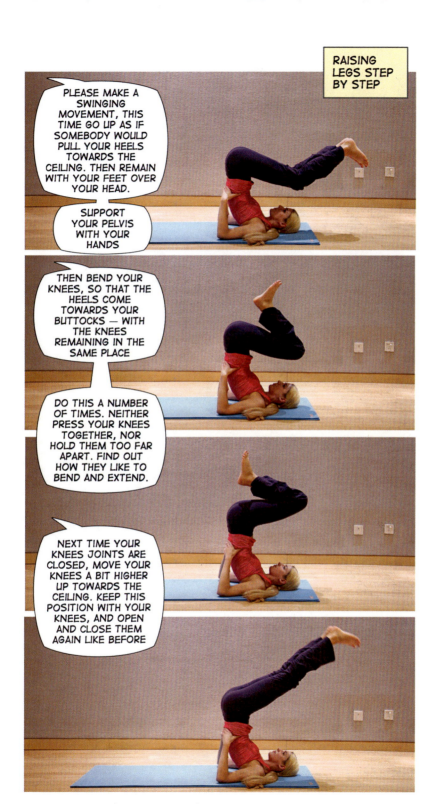

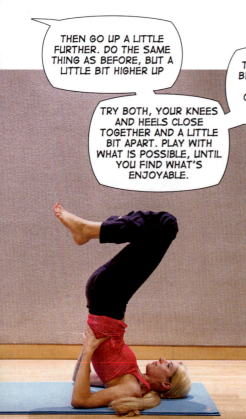
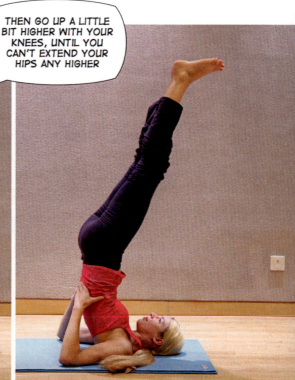
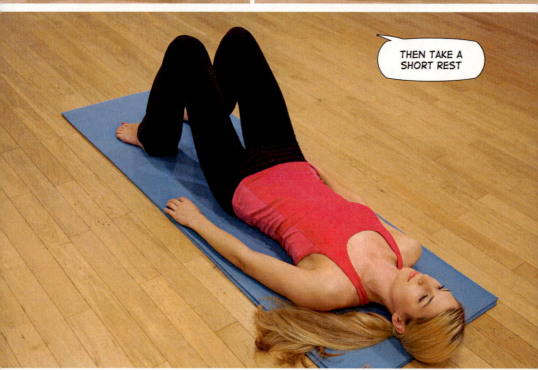

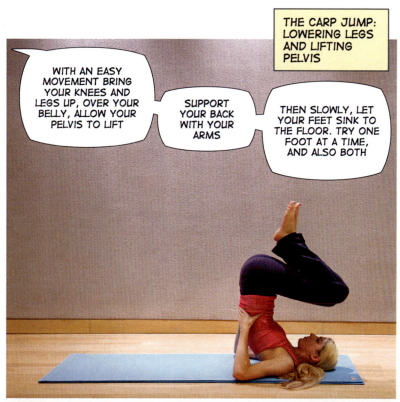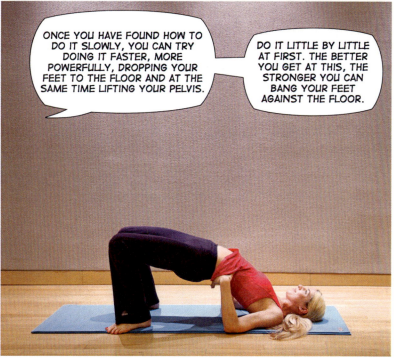

> PUTTING IT ALL
> TOGETHER

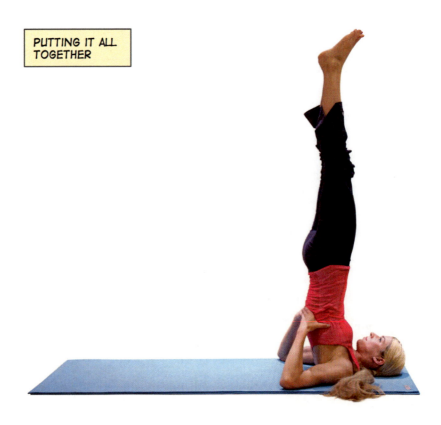

Learn and explore

Learning and copying are not the same actions, yet the former is often mistaken for the latter. Students are required to learn things by heart, when in truth this means to merely copy facts into their brains. In the process of copying there's always a master to copy from, and the copy should ideally look like the master. Now, where is the learning?

A short imaginary journey: you go on holiday to a new place. At first the whole area will be unknown to you. You will ask people where you can withdraw money, where to buy stuff, what kind of transportation is available, what museum or restaurant is important and interesting to go to, and so on. It's an exploration.

By the time a week has past you will know that area. You will know all these things. You will know what you like and what you don't like about this place. You will know whether or not you want to return for another holiday and what to expect. You will know what you missed out on and what you would like to explore further.

You have become proficient in knowing the area via your experience. Now, can this type of learning be transferred into other areas of life? Maybe it doesn't matter whether it's a new town, or a new sport, or a new dish you want to cook, or a language you want to learn. Learning is always an exploration and a transition from a state of not knowing anything – to being proficient, or even being an expert.

The explore movement on ones own is a key study point in Feldenkrais classes. Once the adult has recovered the original „explorer spirit" that children have, this spirit can be applied to other areas. It is a vital skill and will make a positive difference in all kinds of learning endeavours. Only when students take the opportunity to learn and explore will their actions become authentic, skillful, and particularly gratifying to themselves, as well as to others.

Less is more, go with easy

Our culture celebrates the idea of pushing the limits. When trying to achieve something, no amount of stress seems to be too much. „Feel the burn", „destroy those legs", „no pain, no gain" are the mantras. Jane Fonda pioneered this philosophy in the 1980s, and while her taped workouts aren't selling any longer, her catch phrases live on.

Pushing yourself to the limits might give you satisfying feelings in sports and working out, but for in the field of somatic learning pushing it won't have the same effect. You might have some short-term success, but as the stress levels drop, so will your gains.

For learning and refining movement, less is more. It's just so much more effective. If any move hurts, stop immediately. That is your body telling you to not do that particular movement. However, if you discover that something feels pleasant, linger there for a while; that is your body telling you that you need that movement.

This will teach you to find where movement is not yet possible, where it is possible, and where it's easy. Go with easy.

Through such exploration it's then possible for your own inner resources to reorganize the whole body to follow the lead of the easy part. No matter how dominant the inflexible, inaccessible part, there's always something that can be done easily. Then, this will open up things that had to be forced before, or have been entirely inaccessible.

Use it or lose it

Whenever we move, there is the chance to notice something about this move, to vary it, do it a bit differently every time, to refine it, to learn more about it, hopefully leading to constant improvement.

There's also the reverse way: to completely submit a move to habits, with each repetition becoming less and less aware of what is happening with this move. With every repetition a bit more of this move is hidden away from being observable; until it becomes a completely automated habit, and we don't even know that we're doing it. This is not something that happens overnight; it takes years to happen. With many of your moves it will happen in time.

For example: a toddler learns how to sit down and get up. Within a few years there will be some adjustments; but usually after that, a person will keep the same way to get up and sit down over the course of his entire life. Few improvements will be made. Furthermore, if this person never behaves in a way that can lead to improvement, over the years this function will become worse and worse. In the long run, stretching, workout, and muscle strengthening will not prevent a person's way from becoming inadequate. The day will arrive when this person will need assistance to get up and sit down. And this is usually not so much due to old age or loss of strength, but due to a loss of skill.

Recovering such a skill can almost feel like a miracle. For example, a student said after a series of lessons „it's so great to be able to put on my socks by myself again". In such cases recovery of function can almost feel like a miracle. However, the Feldenkrais Method provides much more. Movements that previously seemed impossible become possible; soon what's possible becomes easy, and easy becomes elegant.

Reduce effort, instead of increasing it

Most people know how to work harder and how to apply more and more effort to try and accomplish something. Take for example a screw top jar that won't open on the first try: on the second try, the common action is to apply more force. If that doesn't help, usually one will try to apply even more force (and righteously so). If a door won't open on the first try, on the second try, one pulls harder. If one doesn't understand what the other is saying, eventually the other will speak louder.

I would like to assert that it is possible to go the other way: to actually reduce effort each time – to do less and less with each try. This may not help with opening a stuck lid on a jar, but it does wonders when learning about oneself and others. Such a reduction of effort is not to be confused with relaxation. Instead, it is the ability to turn down the internal „noise level" that comes with great effort, and feel a movement more sensitively each time. This ability will be the basis for making more refined moves and discriminating among them.

Being able to reduce effort will result in a highly refined ability to perceive subtle sensations and motor feedback from the body. This, in turn, is necessary to being able to perform delicate movement.

Spiralling to sit, a classic 4-points lesson

Anyone attending Feldenkrais classes on a regular basis will sooner or later encounter a variant of the 4 points theme. It's just as common as the flexion-extension lessons displayed in previous chapters. There's dozens of these 4 points lessons. They offer a wide variety of movements (including crawling), but most of them have one movement in common: they deal with coming from standing (or sitting on a chair) to sitting on the floor (and up again), from sitting on the floor to lying down (and up again), all in one fluid, spiralling motion.

Kim Wise, Scientist (Anatomy Major), Registered Physiotherapist, Certified Feldenkrais Practitioner and Movement Intelligence teacher, based on the Coffs Coast, NSW Australia, writes: „Every joint in the bodies of vertebrates are not straight, they are curved. An arc exists. When in mathematics we add one bone to another into the bipedal form through arcs, we form a spiral when relating intelligently to gravity. This was/is the beginning of all things as is recorded in the shapes of shells, ferns and many flowers amongst the myriad of forms that reveal the organic nature of the spiral.So, to learn to stand and sit from either a chair or from the floor in a spiral is so much easier, fluid, organic and natural for the human form through the co-ordination of action of the movement in the arcs of movement, not through the mental image of straight lines. This possibility could free the Western World. The spiral of course includes our DNA and with that our evolution."

As people become older or injured, their practice of doing these beautiful spiralling movements usually worsens, until they stop doing them altogether; and thus they lose much of their quality of life. This type of limitation is completely unnecessary — and here you have a remedy. Be kind, be curious, stay hungry, practice often, and include these movements in your everyday life. Or, if sitting on the floor is something you do rather infrequently, briefly practice this lesson once in a while, maybe once a fortnight. Doing so, you will feel unfettered.

Now, please come to your place, we start in standing.

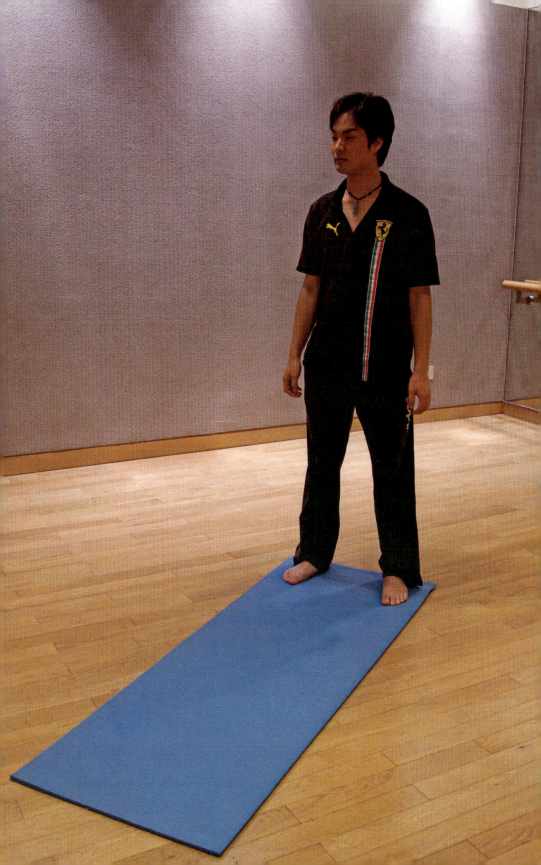

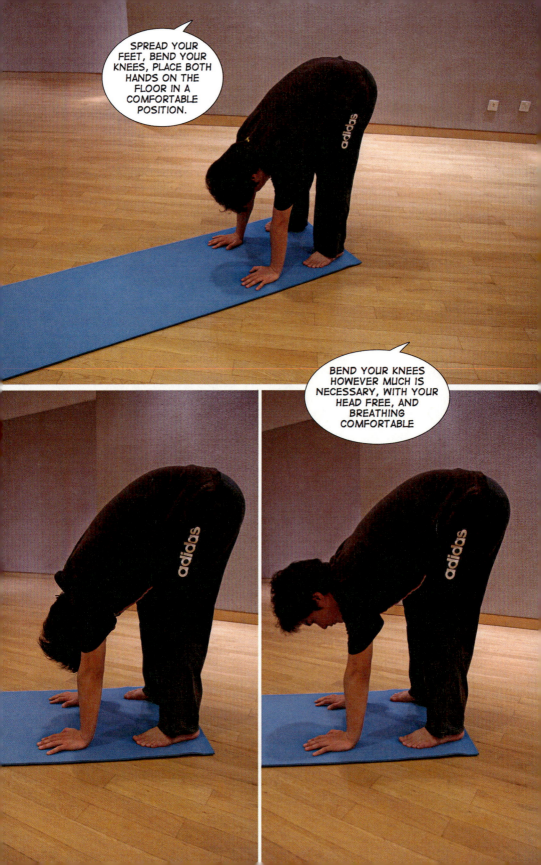

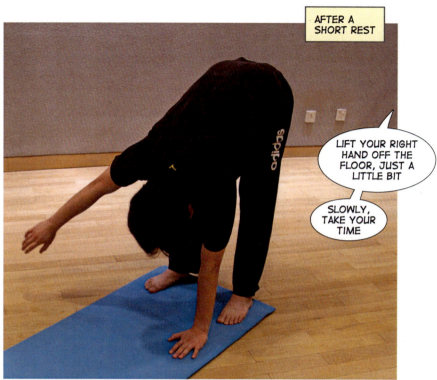
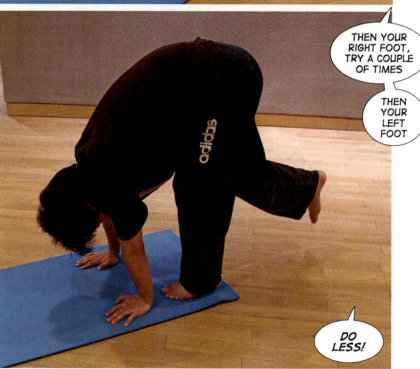

While Feldenkrais practitioners guide their students through Feldenkrais lessons, students are free to focus entirely on HOW to do the lesson, to immerse themselves, to fully be in the present and explore the details at hand. They hardly need to concentrate on the WHAT. However, even though Feldenkrais lessons are always a pliant, lively interaction between practitioner and students, there always is a lesson structure. For this classic 4-points lesson the bare-bones structure looks as follows.

It would have been too much to fit all that text into little speech bubbles, that's why this full page spread is used. For students who like to keep track of sources, this lesson is partly similar to „Alexander Yanai #432: Four points, introduction".

1. In standing: spread your feet, bend your knees, place both hands on the floor. Bend your knees and use your hip joints to be able to touch the floor with your hands. Don't round your back too much. Distribute your wait on all fours. Wait a bit, enjoy the feels, then come up again to standing. Maybe you want to do just this every day.
2. Return to standing on your 4-points. (a) Lift your right hand from the floor and return it to the floor. Do each of the following moves a number of times. (b) Lift your left hand, do not lift high. (c) Lift both hands at the same time and then lean on both of them again. (d) Lift just your right foot a bit. (e) Please lie on your back and rest for a moment.
3. Return to standing on your 4-points. (a) Lift your left foot. Instead of lifting with power, shift your weight, move your pelvis and head, this way it will be very easy (b) Alternate between lifting your right foot and your left foot. (c) Lift both hands. (d) Hop with both feet, then with both hands. Alternate. Be specific with your four points, return hands and feet to the same places. (e) Please lie on your back and rest for a moment.
4. Return to standing on your 4-points. (a) Lift your right hand and right foot together. (b) Lift your left hand and left foot. (c) Alternate between lifting right side and left side. (d) Please lie on your back and rest for a moment.
5. Return to standing on your 4-points. (a) This time lift your right foot and left hand. (b) Lift your left foot and right hand. (c) Lift once your

ght hand and left foot and once the left hand and right foot. (d) Please lie on your back and rest for a moment.

6. Return to standing on your 4-points. (a) Try all the movements you have done so far again. (b) Please lie on your back and rest for a moment.
7. Return to standing on your 4-points. (a) Lift your right leg a bit. Bend it in the knee and turn the pelvis such that it will be possible to sit on the floor and return to all fours. Pass your right knee in between your left hand and left foot. Do this a number of times until it simply is one movement. (b) Do this with and without lifting your hands. (c) Please lie on your back and rest for a moment.
8. Return to standing on your 4-points. (a) Do the same thing with your left knee, sit to the other side. (b) Please lie on your back and rest for a moment.
9. Return to standing on your 4-points. (a) Try to go down once to the right and once to the left side. Lift the foot from the floor each time. (b) As you become better and faster at this movement, change over your feet in the air with a hop. This can be done very quickly. (c) Please lie on your back and rest for a moment.
10. Return to standing on your 4-points. (a) Pass the right knee in between the left foot and left hand as before. This time, lift the left hand from the floor when coming to sit. Lift it and turn completely to the side, looking to the left. Do this many times. (b) Try to turn to the right side. (c) Please lie on your back and rest for a moment.
11. Return to standing on your 4-points. (a) Again alternate between sitting to the left and sitting to the right. (b) Do it faster and faster, change with a hop. (c) Come up to standing, and when you do so, bring your eyes level to the horizon and rise with grace, with a straight torso, like in a Chinese squat or Olympic lift. Don't let your head hang like a broken-hearted teenager would.

Stand for a moment. Try to bend and touch the floor. You will see that, if you pay attention, to get up like this from the floor and to sit down like this to the floor, it's very easy.

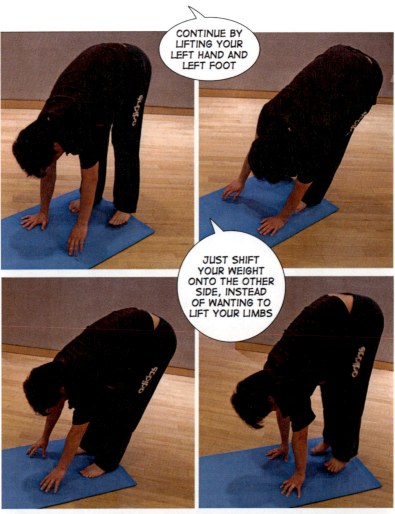
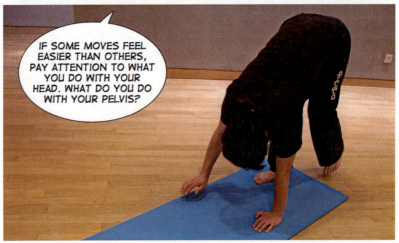

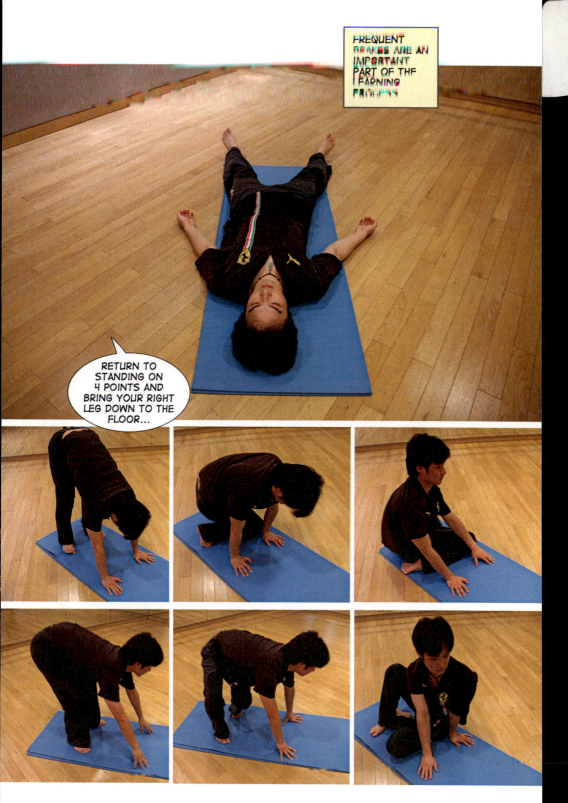

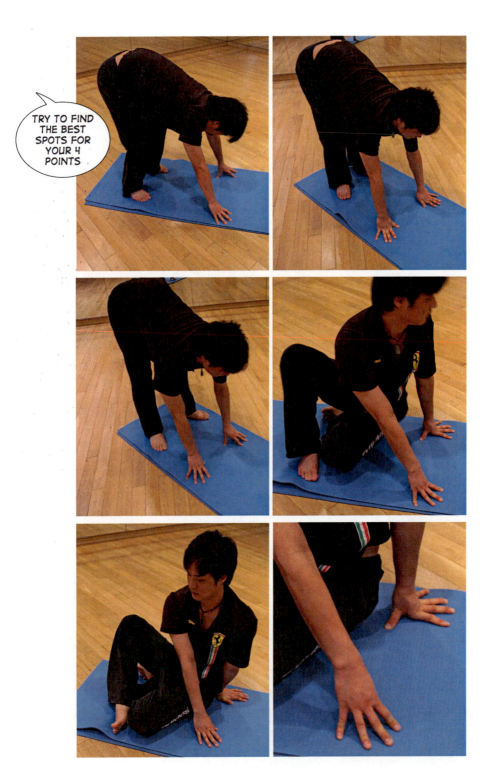

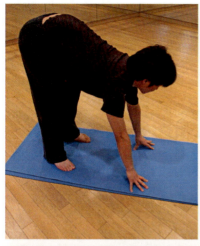
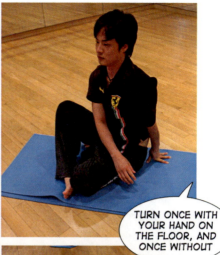

PLEASE
SLOWLY,
SIT UP AND
THEN
GET UP

At the end of a Feldenkrais lesson the practitioner will ask you to get up to standing. „All the world's a stage", says William Shakespeare, „as within, so without" Hermes Trismegistus, „feel how it is and walk a bit" some Feldenkrais practitioners. Whatever it is for you, enjoy the good feelings and then go and do what you do, whatever it is you want to do in your life.

Who created this book?

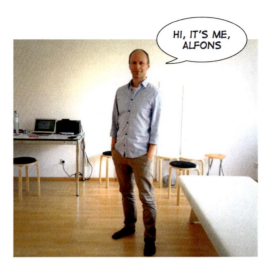

Alfons Grabher is a Guild Certified Feldenkrais Practitioner^{CM} born in 1974 in Vienna, Austria, Europe. He also is a graduate Engineer (University of Applied Sciences, Vienna), specialized in Biomedical Engineering and has worked for over a decade as Software Engineer and Consultant. In 2008 he moved to Shanghai, China to explore more about human life. In 2011 he returned to Austria to set up a professional Feldenkrais practice. His hobbies include publishing free Feldenkrais class recordings (in German language), writing, and making youtube videos.

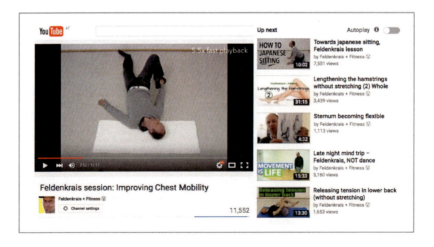

Made in United States
North Haven, CT
23 October 2021